MENO-MOR

Rituals, Spells and Natural Remedies for Peri, Mid, and Postmenopausal Women

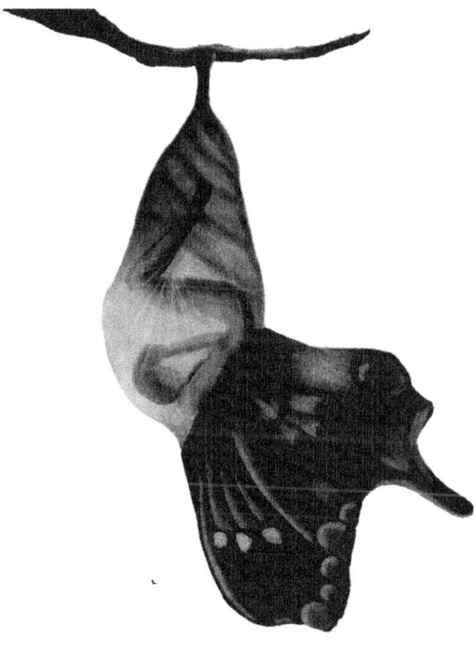

Vanessa Nixon

Traditional Naturopath

Herbs of Grace Press
Centralia, Washington

Meno-Morphosis
Rituals, Spells & Natural Remedies for Peri-Mid-Post Menopausal Women
ISBN 979-8-9870027-0-4
Author Photo by Manon Sund-Kusters
Cover illustration by Ezme Lambert
Cover and Interior Book Design by Cheakina

Library of Congress Control Number: 2022920330

HERBS OF GRACE PRESS

Table of Contents

Medical Disclaimer

All information in this book is based on the personal experiences and education of the author, as well as other health care professionals. It is shared with the understanding that you accept full responsibility for your own health and well being. The results of any suggestions in this book cannot be guaranteed. The author and publisher are not responsible for any adverse effects or consequences resulting from the use of anything included in this book.

Dedication/Acknowledgments

This book is dedicated to my children, who have been the greatest teachers in my life.

Maleah, Scarlet and Isabel, you have taught me how to love and support another human being completely and unconditionally. The honor of being your mother is the greatest gift I have ever received.

I would like to acknowledge all of the incredible people who assisted in the birthing of this book:

My first mentor in natural living, the herbalist Cascade Anderson Geller; Donna Eden, who graciously allowed me to share aspects of her work in these pages; Donna Earnest, whose homeopathic expertise and mentoring have been unquestionably valuable to my work, Ruby Sowder, belly dance teacher extraordinaire; Jessica Hadari, my business mentor; Rosemary Gladstar, Susun Weed and Aviva Romm, whose leadership in the world of herbal medicine and women's health has been inspirational; Jeanne Sullivan Billeci, Meloney Hudson, Vivien Monroe and Veronica Monet for their ongoing support and encouragement; the fabulous and incomparable Cynthia Gregory, without whom this book would not have taken form; my parents, Jim and Joyce Nixon, for their constant support; and finally Thyron Heyward for his love,encouragement and patience.

Introduction

In a span of two years, I turned fifty, went through menopause, got divorced after eighteen years of marriage, moved to a new city, helped two of my daughters move out on their own, bought my first house by myself, restarted my business after years of putting it on the side burner to take care of my children and started dating for the first time in twenty-five years as a postmenopausal woman!

While it was really overwhelming and painful at times, I see now my experiences provided me with the opportunity to create something new in almost every area of my life. I found that I can create this next chapter of my life and step into my power. I can bring my gifts out into the world in alignment with my desires, passions, gifts, wisdom and in the flow of wellness, health and vitality.

I never expected that the most intense challenges of my life would lead me to feel so empowered, so energized and so confident in who I am ...

Who I truly am ...someone I was not encouraged to be before but who I discovered in that two-year crucible. And to come out of that feeling so confident in my ability to tap into my inner wisdom ... to heal myself, my family and my clients is truly magical. And I want that transformation for you too!

As a traditional naturopath, I love helping empower other women to take ownership of their health. I know that if I can tap into my intuition and my inner healer, I can help others to do the same. I am passionate about supporting women to thrive during midlife, using nature as their guide, so they can make this the most vibrant and impactful phase of their lives, through natural health, natural movement and natural beauty.

Do Any of these Sound Familiar?

"Hot flashes … will they ever end?!"

"Sometimes my mood swings are so intense, I don't even recognize myself anymore!"

"I can't even concentrate these days…I feel like I'm losing my mind!"

Can you relate to any of these and worry that it's the new normal you have to tolerate?

The truth is, change can be challenging, but it doesn't have to be painful. And at the end of the process you can come out of the chrysalis expressing your full power and beauty.

But first it helps to have awareness of why you're feeling this way, and to know you are not alone. Did you know that millions of women suffer from menopause-related symptoms such as:

- weight gain
- hot flashes
- night sweats
- mood swings
- brain fog
- memory issues
- low energy
- vaginal dryness

- low libido
- heart palpitations
- muscle and bone loss
- insomnia

They spend years going from doctor to doctor, taking prescription drugs and suffering endless side effects without ever finding the relief they are seeking. Can you relate to that?

In a recent survey I conducted with women just like you, between the ages of thirty-five and sixty-five, the number one desire they have is to feel a sense of wellness, health and vitality and to have confidence in knowing how to achieve it.

That led me to identify **six keys that every woman in midlife needs,** to be able to create consistent wellness rituals, start reducing menopause symptoms using natural methods and learn how to make this the most powerful phase of their life, while feeling sexy, vibrant and focused. You're going to learn those keys in this book!

My Journey

My journey in natural healing began almost thirty years ago …

I had been struggling with chronic, recurring bouts of bronchitis for years. From the age of fifteen to twenty-one, I had been on a downward spiral of illness. I caught every cold that came around and each time, it went deep into my chest and developed into bronchitis. I still remember waking up every morning after a scant few hours of sleep, coughing until my sides ached, my ribs felt bruised and I was too weak to move. As a teenager, one of my worst fears was having a coughing attack in the middle of class and having to rush out of the room with my eyes streaming, barely being able to catch my breath between coughs and ending up in the bathroom, my chest racked with pain and my coughing turning to retching. I had been given all the conventional treatments, including multiple rounds of antibiotics on a regular basis and codeine cough syrups, but my health was continuing to decline.

In my early twenties, my friend David noticed that I was taking antibiotics every day and asked why. When I told him my story, he asked me a question nobody had ever asked me before.

"Is it working?"

I had never thought to ask myself that question … and now that I pondered it, I realized that, no, it was not working. And, that sparked a series of other questions in my mind …

If this is not working, is there another option?

Is there more than one option?

If so, what are they?

As the daughter of a nurse, I had been pretty deeply entrenched in the conventional medical model growing up and I had no idea there were other methods of health care.

That one question – Is it working? – opened my mind to the idea of other possibilities and for the first time in many years, I had hope that things could be different.

David mentioned that when he got sick, he often went to see an herbalist and asked if I would like to be introduced to her. I had never even heard of herbal medicine before and was intrigued. Within a few weeks, I was sick yet again and decided to take him up on his offer. I went to see his herbalist and she gave me an herbal remedy formulated for respiratory illness. To my delight and amazement, what had previously taken me eight weeks to recover from … taking the herbal formula, I recovered in two weeks' time! And, even more amazingly, the recurrences became less and less frequent until bronchitis became a thing of the past for me.

That did it!

I was hooked.

I began my journey of creating a natural lifestyle and maintaining true wellness for myself no matter what health challenges I faced. And, at the time of writing, I have not had a bout of bronchitis in almost twenty years!

To give you a brief overview of this journey:

- In my twenties, I rebuilt my health after suffering from chronic respiratory illness for almost seven years.
- In my late twenties and early thirties I incorporated teachings and trainings from a multitude of natural modalities to up-level my health as well as that of my growing family.
- In my thirties and forties I raised three healthy daughters exclusively with natural medicine. From meals of foraged wild greens and eggs and vegetables we raised ourselves, to oral care tonics, to earache and sunburn relief, you name it; I had a remedy and my girls were my home lab!
- AND, over the last ten years, I have been teaching and mentoring other women to do the same. I've helped my clients overcome mood swings, digestive issues, weight challenges and even chronic illness.

As I am now navigating the waters of the menopausal journey myself, I can relate to my clients on a deep, personal level and bring them solutions that I know will work because I've experienced them in my own life.

I'd like to give you the keys to harness the power of nature to increase your health, grow your confidence in taking charge of your own wellness and elevate your life by connecting with your intuitive magic.

Let me show you how I created radiant health in body, mind and spirit through the healing remedies that nature provides ...

Even though I came into menopause having had three decades of practicing optimal nutrition, herbal medicine, flower essences and homeopathy to raise my general level of health to an incredibly high standard, I still experienced some unexpected challenges when I hit menopause.

After healing myself of my chronic respiratory illnesses in my early twenties, I began devouring every book I could get my hands on that might help me to understand why the herbal remedy I took was so effective. I started a course of self-study in herbalism with the works of Susun Weed and Rosemary Gladstar, among many others, and soon enrolled in official herbal studies courses with well-renowned herbalist Cascade Anderson Geller. That led me to understand that what I had been eating all my life needed close inspection ... which led me to other natural modalities ... and still other natural healing methods. Soon, I was experiencing such a different lifestyle that I hardly remembered what it had been like to suffer as I had for so many years. My energy levels, productivity, creativity and joy were at such a high level on a daily basis that my old life seemed like it had been lived by someone else. Sure, I still came down with a cold every once in a while, but the difference was that now, I had the confidence and skills to heal myself quickly and the wisdom to listen to what my body needed in the moment.

So, when I entered the waters of perimenopause, I expected smooth sailing ...

Ha! If only I knew then what I know now!

Mood swings and emotional outbursts really caught me by surprise. Even though I had always had "the gift of tears" (as a good friend and client once called it), I found myself crying at the most inopportune moments. Even though I had always considered myself to be extremely patient, I found it was wearing thin. And, even though I was confident in my ability to manage my personal relationships with relative ease, I found myself in a marriage that was hurtful, unsupportive and at a dead end. I found myself living with a constant knot in my belly, not knowing where I was going to end up or how to make sure my children were not traumatized in the process.

And, as I mentioned earlier, my marriage of over eighteen years did end in divorce, I moved to a new town, bought my own home by myself for the first time, experienced my eldest two daughters moving out on their own, began to focus on my career for the first time after taking twenty years off to raise my children AND started dating for the first time in twenty-five years as a menopausal woman!

I was experiencing so many changes in my life, all at the same time! And, believe me when I say that these years were definitely the most challenging of my life!

But there was one thing that made the difference for me and helped me start to turn everything around …

When things were the most difficult and I was struggling the most …

I remembered that I had resources …

I had tools and techniques …

and most of all …

I had support.

I had women friends and mentors I could lean on, who provided safe spaces for me to process what I was going through so I could move forward.

I had my education in nutrition, herbal medicine, flower essences, homeopathy, aromatherapy and reflexology to lean on.

And, I had a connection to my inner healer, my intuition, my innate wisdom to know what my mind, body and soul needed to move me forward and elevate my life to a new level, a new place of health, fulfillment and abundance I had never experienced before!

So I can honestly say that I've been through the initiation!

I've been through the fire and I came out on the other side!

And I can see that every piece of what I just shared with you has been an opportunity. An opportunity for growth, an opportunity for healing and an opportunity to share my gifts with others and truly make a positive difference in their lives!

And, the best part of this entire journey is that I know if I can do this ... I can help other women do the same.

Another thing that I discovered along the way though, was that many women, if not most women, have similar experiences as they journey through the transitions from perimenopause, through menopause and into post-menopause. But most of them have not had the privilege of coming into this phase of life with a high level of health to begin with, or with a support system to draw from, so they are often really suffering. The symptoms they experience sometimes keep them in bed all day, lead them to withdraw from their social life, and worsen their connection to their own bodies and minds. Some women have even confided that they feel like they are losing their minds! They fear for their health, their future and they don't know where to turn.

Jacqui's Journey Part I

When Jacqui came to me, she had been experiencing a plethora of midlife symptoms including worsening PMS (feeling like Jekyll and Hyde throughout her cycles), waning libido, fatigue, irritability, mental confusion, brain fog and memory loss. As a trained health-care professional herself, she had seen many practitioners and was quite tired of, as she said, "being fobbed off left and right by the medical model."

After a few months of working together she had a big aha moment … She had felt like her life was one big jigsaw puzzle with a piece missing. In our work together, through movement, natural remedies and creating self-loving rituals, that missing piece suddenly fell into place and in her words, "I was not experiencing the terrible all-encompassing brain fog now that I had learned to support my mind and body with nutrition and herbal support … I now can feel a whole new sense of purpose just being me … who and how I am. And this is all fun!"

If this is possible for Jacqui, then it's possible for you. Let me help you initiate your Meno-Morphosis now.

Chapter 1

The Myths, Magic, and Meaning of Menopause

Women often experience fear, frustration, struggle, and overwhelm during the metamorphosis of menopause. Two of the reasons we can feel so frustrated and overwhelmed during this phase of life are lack of information and misinformation.

- Lack of information because there is a taboo around talking about menopause in our society.
- Misinformation because of the way our society has conditioned us to feel about menopause.

In fact one of the most glaring examples of the lack of information surrounding "the change" is that so many women are not even sure exactly what menopause is! Most women I speak with are questioning if they might be in menopause … what perimenopause is … and have never even thought or heard the term post-menopause. A lot of women haven't talked much about it and believe that at some point, their menstrual cycles will stop and then they will be in menopause for the rest of their life. Do any of these perspectives apply to you? If so, you are not alone.

In a recent poll conducted by GenM, a UK organization created to provide better support to all those in menopause, they found that 75 percent of women still feel the topic cannot even be openly discussed.

Which Menopause Phase are You In?

Here are the technical definitions of the terms used to refer to the menopausal journey and what is powerful about them, as represented by three iconic Hindu goddesses:

- Perimenopause: The time in a woman's life when physiological changes occur that begin the transition to menopause. Perimenopause means "around menopause" and refers to the time during which your body makes the natural transition to menopause, marking the end of the reproductive years. Some people refer to this phase as the "menopausal transition."
- Menopause: Menopause is a point in time twelve months after a woman's last period. Menopause is the time that marks the end of your menstrual cycles. It's diagnosed after you've gone twelve consecutive months without a menstrual period.
- Post-menopause: This is the time after menopause. Technically, a woman is postmenopausal from the day menopause occurs until the end of her life.

- Another term that is quite confusing is pre-menopause, which just means anytime in a woman's life before menopause (whether physiological changes are occurring or not).

Welcoming Goddess Wisdom

Now that we understand these terms, let's move on to menopause myths … But before we do, I'd love to introduce you to three goddesses who symbolize the three stages of the menopausal journey we just defined, to help you start seeing the wisdom in each phase. In the Hindu tradition, there are ten wisdom goddesses (or Mahavidyas) who can help guide us through the natural rhythms of life. These three are linked to the menopausal phase of life:

- Bagalamukhi is associated with perimenopause. She is able to stop a person in their tracks, paralyzing them. She embodies the step into the unknown and a turning inward of the consciousness.
- Bhairavi is the guardian over menopause. She is the warrior goddess, who gifts the qualities of clarity and fearlessness to us in the time of reevaluation that is offered to us at this phase of life.
- Dhumavati is the grandmother goddess who stands over the final period of postmenopausal wisdom. She teaches us to be free from external attachments and how to accept the impermanence of life so we can focus on what truly matters.

There are many myths and misconceptions surrounding menopause that we have been conditioned to believe … and since menopause is such a taboo subject, there is little frank discussion happening to dismiss them. I'd like to talk about the top three myths of menopause and then reframe them. Let's bust these myths!

Top 3 Menopause Myths

1. Myth Number One: Menopause = Death

Menopause equals death? This sounds extreme and dire, and not rational, but it is ingrained in our minds nonetheless.

In past centuries, women often didn't live past menopause. Statistics show that the average lifespan a century ago in the US for a woman was fifty-three years. Two centuries ago, it was only thirty-five years!

If you lived through menopause, you had lived to a ripe old age and were practically at death's door.

Now for the reframe …

We know this myth isn't literally true. We know that menopause does not literally equal death. However, the notion remains in our consciousness and that is why we need to address it and dismiss it with new information.

Today, the life expectancy for women in the US is eighty-one years and in other parts of the world it is even higher. The centenarian population (population of people living over one hundred years) is projected to grow eightfold in the next few decades. Eighty percent of centenarians are women! What that means is that many of us can expect to live more years after menopause than we did before menopause. Some of us will even live more decades after menopause than we did before that transition.

So not only does menopause not equal death, it is only the midway point of life for most of us and for some of us not even that!

2. Myth Number Two: Menopause is a Medical Disease

The unfortunate reality is that our medical field has framed menopause as a deficiency disease. Menopause is thought of as a state of illness in which there is a deficiency of hormones in a woman's body. We are made to believe that in menopause we are unhealthy, needing treatment, needing drugs, needing surgery. We are told that menopause is a medical condition that needs medical treatment to be resolved.

Now for the reframe ...

In truth, menopause is a natural and normal phase of life for a woman to go through.

It is not a deficiency of hormones. It does not require medical treatment. This is what our bodies are supposed to do at this point in life. This is the natural cycle that women flow through during this phase of their lives. All women who live past the reproductive stage of life are meant to go through menopause.

I want to challenge you to look at it as an honor that you get to experience ...

The fact that, in this century, we have the opportunity to go through menopause and live a vibrant long life is a gift that most women previously were not given ...

3. Myth Number Three: Life will Never be the Same

We are conditioned to believe that once we go through "the change," we will be suffering through extreme physical, mental and emotional symptoms. That there is nothing we can do about it. We will suffer hot flashes, weight gain, low sex drive, memory loss, invisibility, sagging and wrinkled skin, and so on. In short, everything is downhill from here. In our culture, youth is revered for its fresh beauty, lively energy and juicy vitality. Once a woman in our culture reaches a certain age … suddenly it is as if she is no longer visible … she disappears … and may sometimes feel as if she is of little consequence. Our conditioning would have us believe that our productive lives are over once our reproductive lives are over.

Now for the reframe …

Actually, in one way, this is not so much of a myth. It's true, your life will not be the same.

But is that a bad thing? The myth is that we must suffer, and our lives will go downhill.

The truth is that, while your life will undoubtedly change, you don't have to suffer.

There are many things you can do if you experience uncomfortable symptoms, but not all women do. In fact, some women sail through this phase of life and experience more joy than ever! Some women love that they no longer have to deal with menstrual periods or the possibility of pregnancy. Many women find that this can be the best time of their lives. In fact, research has recently determined that the most productive decades of life are from the fifties through the eighties!

This is the bottom line – what I want you to feel, deep down inside:

- This can be the most empowered, vital and healthy phase of your life.
- This can absolutely be the most powerful, impactful and fulfilling time of your life.
- This can be the chapter of your life when you really get to create the life of your dreams.

Can you feel that?

If you aren't feeling it quite yet … can you imagine it?

Can you hold it as a real possibility for you?

You may be feeling like you have no idea how to start changing your experience of midlife or menopause … You may be thinking … how can I possibly feel healthy or vibrant?

I get it … this has been ingrained into us by our culture … but it doesn't have to be that way. It can be simpler than you think. You may feel overwhelmed by the thought of all the changes you think you have to make. I know how that feels … but taking things step by step can make things so much easier than you might imagine. This is one of the things I love to help my clients with, so they feel empowered!

Take a Meno-Moment

Right now I'd like you to take a deep breath and spend a moment grounding yourself with me.

Close your eyes.
Sit comfortably.
Take a few deep belly breaths.
Really start to feel in your body the feeling that this phase of life can be easy.
Being healthy and happy during midlife can be simple.
This really can happen for you.
This can absolutely be the most powerful, impactful and fulfilling time of your life.
Pay attention to how that feels in your body.
Breathe it into your body.
Release the old myths.
Release the misconceptions you've held.
Breathe in your power, your health and your vitality.
Breathe in the truth.
Take a couple more breaths deep into your belly.
When you're ready, open your eyes.

How was that for you? Do you feel it? Can you at least imagine your life like that?

The last thing I want to suggest before you move forward is to take the Meno-Morphosis Midlife Assessment (https://forms.gle/1Q6hgA2SHddcX8ps6). Completing this assessment is the place where you start your Vibrant Midlife Goddess Plan. This will give you a clear picture of where you are now and where you need to go to reach your goals. This is the beginning of how you will create consistent rituals, start reducing menopause symptoms using natural methods and learn how to make this the most powerful phase of your life, while feeling energized, vibrant and focused!

Chapter 2

Menopause Is Your Spiritual Initiation

To create any sort of lasting change in your life, one of the most important things to begin with is your mindset. Gustavo Razzetti writes in *Psychology Today,* "Your success and happiness depend on your mindset. What you think, you become. Our mindset affects how we see the world. If yours is distorted, so will be the way you see yourself and others. Our beliefs and thoughts shape the way we behave, even if we don't realize it. Developing the right mindset is crucial to succeeding in life."

Here are a few mindset principles that will help you get the most out of this book. They will help you focus on your personal health goals and help you integrate what you learn in this book into your life.

When you are able to do that, you can create consistent rituals …

You can start reducing menopause symptoms using natural methods …

You can learn how to make this the most powerful phase of your life …

And, you can do it while feeling sexy, vibrant and focused!

That's why you're here and that's what I want for you.

The truth is, this can just be just another self-help book, like many you've invested in before. You read it, get inspired, then put it on your bookshelf and forget about it.

Or this can be a life-changing transformation for you. If you are able to allow self-love, self-care, and self-compassion, then real change can occur. Only you can make the difference. Maybe you've been trying to improve your health for a long time now and you haven't seen results.

Maybe you're wondering if this time will be any different … I'm here to remind you that this time, it CAN be different. I'm inviting you to set the intention … right now … to make it different.

I'm taking a stand for you right now. You've invested your money, time, and energy in reading this book because you're ready to make a positive change in your life. You're ready to regain your health. You're ready to step into the next phase of your life as the empowered, wise goddess that you truly are. Your success in this is only limited by what you do next.

My hope is that you will set your intention for fully participating and making the most of this experience. I can't do that for you. I'm here to give you the information that you need and support you in every way that I can, but it's up to you to take that information and implement it, integrate it and make it part of your lifestyle.

One of the best ways to do that is to remind yourself why you decided to focus on improving your health in the first place.

What are your reasons?

What's your biggest why?

Is it because insomnia leaves you so tired that you lack the energy to focus on your job, spend enough time with your children, or give your best to your relationship?

Is it because your hot flashes interrupt you day and night, making you feel so miserable that you snap at your coworkers, children, and spouse and negatively affect your ability to accomplish the things you need to get done? Or is it because mood swings affect you so intensely that you're afraid you're damaging the relationships in your life that are so important to you? Many women I speak with are secretly afraid that they are going crazy at this time in their lives and they are afraid for their future.

No matter what it is for you, spend a few minutes right now thinking about your biggest why:

Why do you need to resolve your menopausal symptoms?

What are they costing you?

What are they preventing you from doing, being or accomplishing in your life?

And why is this important to you?

Think about why this is important in your personal life.

And, then think about why this is important in an altruistic way. What are you not able to give to the world because of where you are right now? What is this situation preventing you from achieving on a larger scale, what dreams do you have, what difference could you make in the world, what impact could you make on others, if only you could overcome this obstacle? I'm asking you to reach really deep right now and identify your biggest whys on a personal level and an altruistic level and write them down.

And, now I'm going to ask you to imagine what your life will look like once these issues are resolved.

How will your relationships improve?

Your work relationships, your relationships with your children, your partner, your family members, your friends? How will your daily life improve?

How will you feel throughout your days when you no longer have to spend all your energy dealing with hot flashes, insomnia, brain fog and mood swings?

What will that look like?

What will that feel like?

What is that worth to you?

Is it worth setting aside thirty minutes or an hour a day to spend on yourself?

Is it worth taking care of yourself, practicing self-care, and integrating lifestyle habits that will help you achieve your goals?

I think it is and I am taking that stand for you today. And, I invite you to take a stand for yourself and fully commit right now.

One of the ways you can do that is to close all your escape hatches. We all have escape hatches. Those little excuses we give ourselves to get out of the work we need to do to improve our lives. The outs we give ourselves. I'm too tired today, I need to attend to other people's needs, it's too much, I'm too overwhelmed … all those "toos."

Or maybe for you, it's something like … Well, it's not that bad after all, I've made some headway, that's enough for now. Or maybe it's … I've tried this before and it didn't work then, or I tried and I just can't do it.

Whatever your escape hatch is … close it. You can do this and it can work for you. If you didn't believe that deep down, you wouldn't be here right now. But you are here, so go all in and close that escape hatch behind you!

Another way to take a stand for yourself and get the most out of this book is to focus on what you can do and not what you can't. It may be tempting to start feeling overloaded with so much information and action steps to take that you tell yourself you can't do it all. When that happens, and let's be real, we all feel overwhelmed at some point when we decide to make changes in our lives, so it will happen, and when it does … remind yourself to only focus on what you can do. Don't think about what you can't do. Remember that there are always things you can do and focus on those things. Then, when you've done those things, and integrated them into your daily life, go back and focus on the next step. Stay focused on what you can do in each moment.

When you feel overwhelmed, remember, this is normal, it's OK to feel this way, everybody does sometimes. And, remind yourself that what you're doing here will not take forever. Perhaps only a few weeks or months. You can do anything for a few weeks. And, what you do here, in these weeks and months, will have such an amazingly positive impact on your health and your life, reaching far into the future, it is so worth it.

You can do this!

Lastly, I want to address one more way that many people prevent themselves from receiving the help that is being offered to them. I hear it all the time. It goes something like this:

"Oh, I already tried that and it didn't work for me."

"I've already heard this information."

"I know this already. "

I lovingly call this the know-it-all syndrome. And, I can say this to you because I've been there before myself. You may have heard some or even much of the information in this book, but it doesn't mean that you know it. Hearing something or trying something doesn't mean you've integrated it. It doesn't mean you know it and it doesn't mean that you've experienced it in the same context as now. Sometimes it takes many experiences with something new before it sinks in and sometimes it just takes hearing it in a new way.

It's true that you may truly know some of what you will be getting in this book, but I encourage you to take the perspective that you are here for a reason; you're hearing it right now because it's what you need to hear and there is a way to experience it in a deeper, more meaningful way.

There's always more to learn about a subject you already know well.

I've been studying and working with natural medicine for decades and I still learn new things literally every day. And, so do you. So, I invite you to embrace the things you already know and then look deeper for a more meaningful understanding of those things you know, while at the same time, taking in the new information as well.

Tapping Into the Wisdom of Your Journey

Your next step is to complete the exercises I have for you here and in the first one, write down your biggest *whys*, close your escape hatches and make your commitment to yourself and your health!

Menopause is Your Spiritual Initiation

WHAT'S YOUR WHY?

Why did you decidedto focus on improving your health in the first place? What are your reasons? What's your biggest why?
Spend a few minutes right now, thinking about your biggest why....
Why do you need to resolve your menopausal symptoms?
What are they costing you?
What are they preventing you from doing, being or accomplishing in your life?
And why is this important to you?
Think about why this is important in your personal life.

And now, think bout why this is important in an altruistic way.
What are you not able to give to the world because of where you are right now?
What is this situation preventing you from achieving on a larger scale,
what dreams do you have, what difference could you make in the world,
what impact could you make on others,
if only you could overcome this obstacle? I'm asking you to reach really deep
right now and identify your biggest why's on an altruistic level and write them down.

And, now I'm going to ask you to imagine what your life will look like once these issues are resolved. How will your relationships improve? Your work relationships, your relationships with your children, your partner, your family members, your friends? How will your daily life improve? How will you feel throughout your days when you no longer have to spend all your energy dealing with hot flashes, insomnia, brain fog and mood swings? What will that look like? What will that feel like?
What is that worth to you? Is it worth setting aside 30 minutes or an hour a day to spend on yourself?

Close all your escape hatches! We all have escape hatches....those little excuses we give ourselves to get out of the work we need to do to improve our lives. The Outs we give ourselves.....I'm too tired today, I need to attend to other people's needs, it's too much, I'm too overwhelmed...all those too's. Or maybe for you, it's something like...well, it's not that bad after all, I've made some headway, that's enough for now. or maybe it's I've tried this before and it didn't work then, or I tried and I just can't do it. Whatever your escape hatch is....close it. Write down your escape hatches and what you're going to do to close them.

VIBRANT MID-LIFE | Revolution

To begin to understand the mystery of hormones, mood, food, and life events, you need to pay attention. By keeping a daily diary, you can learn to read the patterns of your body and its consequences. You can copy and print out this Food Mood Journal if you like. This is one of the tools you'll be using to track your progress. It has space to track your daily food/beverage intake as well as mood/emotions, events, menstrual changes, and so on.

It's important to make a few minutes in your schedule every day to sit and reflect on your activities and why they're important, as well as how they change over time and how this affects you. It's the only way to see correlations between what you are doing and the effects it has on you, as well as the changes you make and what effect they have on you. You can only do this if you track it.

So, make the decision right now to commit to this small but highly effective technique.

FOOD MOOD JOURNAL

DATE	
BREAKFAST	
BRUSH TEETH/SHOWER	
SNACK	
LUNCH	
SNACK	
DINNER	
SNACK	
EXERCISE	
SLEEP & DREAMS	
SUPPLEMENTS/HERBS MEDICATION	
WATER	
SYMPTOMS	
SITTING	
MENSTRUAL CYCLE DAY, BLEEDING, SYMPTOMS	
MOOD/EMOTIONS	
MEDITATION	
ENERGY MEDICINE	
MOON PHASE	
EVENTS	

VIBRANT MID-LIFE Revolution

Magical Midlife Reset

Another reset that is critical to undertake is the mindset around the conditioning we have had about midlife and menopause. In the previous chapter we talked about some of the myths surrounding menopause and then reframed them. I'd like to go a little deeper now.

We discussed how one of the most common misconceptions around menopause is how it is so closely associated in our collective consciousness with death. In the year 1900 (which is only a little over one hundred years ago), white women were expected to live until age forty-nine. And in that same year, African American women were only expected to live until age thirty-four! So, this concept that menopause is associated with death is still lodged in our ancestral memory. Even though we know, intellectually, that the life expectancy for a woman now is in her eighties, that memory of not living past menopause is like an emotional veil that has been placed in our subconscious around the menopausal phase of life.

We still feel it …

We subconsciously still believe it …

And it informs the decisions we make and how we move in the world.

Reframing this belief is key to catapulting our ability to heal ourselves and create vibrant health in this chapter of our lives!

Another part of this that needs a little unpacking is that, in one way, menopause does equal death. It is the death of our reproductive years. It marks the end of the period of time when a woman can potentially bear a child. And, whether a woman already has children and does not want more, has children and would love to have more, wanted children but never had them or never wanted to bear children at all … the finality of not being able to potentially bear a child anymore … having that possibility disappear … can feel like an incredibly intense loss.

And that loss needs to be addressed.

The emotions that come up around this need to be allowed.

We need to give ourselves permission to grieve this death, so that we can move on to the magical opportunities that await us.

We also reframed the misconception that everything is going to go downhill after menopause and we will suffer increasingly disruptive symptoms for the rest of our lives. And how, actually for many women, menopause is a breeze and the most vital time of their lives.

I'd like to briefly introduce the idea here that the symptoms we might experience during the transition of menopause can be reframed as an opportunity to uncover parts of ourselves we may not have had the time, energy or space to delve into earlier in our lives. We have the opportunity to pause during meno-pause and really listen to the messages our bodies are sending us, really tune in to our intuition and resolve issues or outdated beliefs that we may still be clinging to.

As with the metamorphosis of the butterfly … sometimes we need to cocoon ourselves and allow the body that we are familiar with to reshape itself and grow the wings we are meant to develop so we can reach new heights.

Menopause as a Spiritual Initiation

Have you heard of this concept? There is so much power in that statement. I first heard this phrase from Kat Codrington, menstrual and menopause mentor (https://www.katecodrington.co.uk/). But what exactly does it mean? I believe it means that this is an opportunity for us to really go deep inside and evaluate our lives and truly consider:

What we've accomplished.

What wisdom we've gained.

How we want to bring that to the world.

How can we step forward in our power.

How can we use our passions and the things we really care about, to help our families, our communities, other women and the world from a place of deep wisdom, in alignment with our own intuition and higher power.

This is the spiritual initiation we are called to step into!

I read in a book that there is an American Indian saying that goes like this:

On her first bleed – a woman MEETS her power

During her bleeding years – she PRACTICES her power

And at menopause – she BECOMES her POWER!

DO you feel it?

Is this something that speaks to you?

Do you know that you have more inside of you that you want to bring into being, that you want to create in this next phase of your life?

As I've mentioned before, our culture does not tend to value the maturing woman. From the way we are made to feel invisible in the workplace to the way our concerns are not heard in the medical office to the way the media portrays older women as no longer desirable or beautiful, it is no wonder menopause is looked at with indifference, dread, and even fear.

It hasn't always been that way though, and it still isn't in many parts of the world. Menopause is no longer synonymous with the end of a woman's life. It is only the midpoint. Most women can look forward to the next half of their life unfolding before them as they go through menopause. Some women will live more years of their life post-menopausal than they did before entering menopause. The stigma of menopause signaling old age and death is no longer valid. We need a new way to think about this phase of life. Or maybe more accurately, we need to look back on how menopause has been experienced and exalted in more traditional cultures around the world.

This is what *Meno-Morphosis* is all about. This is the time for us to step into our power and use all the wisdom we've accumulated up till now and share it with the world.

In fact, Amanda McQuade Crawford said it very well in her book *The Natural Menopause Handbook:*

> *"After a temporary period of trial, whether mild or intense, every woman can enter the second half of her life with a wisdom and dignity no maiden can match."*

In several Asian cultures, menopause is known as the second spring. It is viewed as the awakening or rebirthing period of a woman's life ... the springtime of the second half of her life. What a refreshing way to look at it, right?

The second spring is our time to refocus on ourselves and our lives and remind ourselves what we are really passionate about. We often become disconnected from our passions after nurturing others for many years of our lives. It's time to start nurturing ourselves. Self-nurture can lead us back to what's really important to us, can fill up our cup, so that we have an overflow to give to others and the world and help us rekindle our desires and passions for who we want to be in the world and what we are here to do what impact we want to make – we need deep nourishment and nurturing of ourselves to bring that to fruition.

In the goddess culture, midlife and menopause are highly revered for the wisdom and knowledge a woman has gained by this time in her life. For example, the goddess Metis is known as the mature goddess archetype of practical wisdom. She represents the woman who uses her intelligence in practical and useful ways and she uses wisdom and skill to make quick and effective decisions. She knows how to mediate confrontational situations and create peace and harmony in her environment, according to Jean Bakula, astrologist.

In recent years in our own culture, there has been a change in the way many people view menopause. A great quote from Margaret Mead goes like this:

"The most creative force in the world is the menopausal woman with zest."

Why does having zest, or for that matter creativity, in the menopausal years matter to our health? Here's what the science says:

A 1998 Gallup survey showed more than 50 percent of US women felt happiest and most fulfilled at this stage of life. And, according to Dr. Mercola, one recent study has linked having a sense of purpose in life to reduced odds of suffering a stroke. More than 450 elderly were included in the study, and underwent annual physical and psychological evaluations until their death. Purpose in Life was judged on a five-point scale, and for every one-point increase in the score, the odds of having a macroscopic infarction (clearly visible stroke damage at autopsy) went down by about 50 percent. In all, those with a strong sense of life purpose were 44 percent less likely to have suffered the kind of major brain tissue damage that drives up your risk of age-related dementia and disability.

Another piece of research in 2008 in the Journal of *Psychological Science in the Public Interest* charted the range of cognition (how well our brains can function) at various ages. They discovered that the potential for high-functioning brain activity peaks in our fifties but remains high until our nineties and functional into the hundreds. However, they also found that the *average* person peaks at thirty and declines to a nonfunctioning state by his or her late eighties. This speaks to the untapped potential that is here for us if we address, nurture and cultivate it.

Dr. Christiane Northrup refers to menopause as *"the mother of all wake-up calls."* I agree. It's time to wake up and get to work on ourselves. But, what does that really mean?

Well, for one thing, it reminds us that our symptoms are messages our body/mind/soul are sending us to address. It gives us more information about our internal environment and it is a conversation we need to pay attention to, to help us become a better version of ourselves.

My friend Jamila White wrote something recently that I feel is befitting this discussion and I'd like to share it with you …

*"Sis, sometimes what you're going through isn't an ordinary struggle. Sometimes it's an *initiation.**

When you feel like you're facing multiple battles on multiple fronts – and you may even feel like you're 'dying' (i.e., the life you created for yourself is falling apart) – you may be going through a Spirit-led initiation. An initiation, once all is said and done, changes how you see yourself and the world around you. It is an incredibly powerful transformation. While it's happening, though, it rocks you to your very core.

The question isn't 'Why is this happening to me?'

The better questions are:

What new level of myself am I being initiated to?

*What am I passing to and what portal am I passing *through*?*

What am I being prepared for?

What blessings am I being uncomfortably stretched for, so that I can expand my capacity to receive?

What parts of me are ready to die off so that I can birth my next level?

What do I need to surrender and release?

What am I learning right now?

*You are being called higher, love. It's like being in a video game and you reach a new level – and the old tools from the previous level don't work here. A new level requires new tools and new energy. It may feel a bit disorienting to be thrust into a new world and discover that none of your old tools (habits, practices) work. Start exploring new tools or new ways of using old tools. The best thing you can do in the middle of an initiation by Spirit is to *not resist.**

Your instinct is usually going to be to fight for control. You aren't in control of this, love.

If something needs to break, let it. If someone needs to leave, let them. If you need to go, go.

ALLOW IT.

Release your grip on struggle. Release your attachment to the outcome. The harder you hold on to what was (or what you hoped was), the more difficult this part of your journey will be. LET GO … Or be dragged.

Your power is in your choice. Whatever shows up in an initiation season, try to observe it without attachment. Sometimes healing work is messy AF. But it's so, so worth it. There is light at the end of this tunnel. And that beautiful light is YOU, sis!

I already see you radiating the light of your newly-initiated self, and – my, my, my – what a sight to behold.

Keep going.

I love you. ~J."

– Jamila White

www.InspiredJamila.com

Wow!

It makes me tear up every time I read it …

Is that on point or what?

Can you relate to that?

I certainly can and I think every woman going through the challenges of midlife can, to some degree. I invite you to go back to this quote whenever you feel overwhelmed by the changes that are occurring in your life and reread it. Reread it as many times as you need to.

The challenges of midlife exist for a reason. Kate Codrington asserts that one of the challenges we have at this time is to confront the unknown and to be able to sit with our grief. It's a time to reexamine our beliefs around aging, to get clear about our values. And, it brings to us the gift of nonnegotiable self-care. And this is one of the reasons our sensitivities tend to increase at this time – psychically, spiritually, physically.

This reminds us once again, our symptoms are messages our body/mind/soul sends to us to address.

This is our initiation.

This is our opportunity to take.

This is what enables us to step into our power and fulfill our calling and to live our bliss (as Joseph Campbell so wisely put it).

"The change" (as menopause has been referred to) is the birth of the wise woman. Women's mysteries teacher Jane Hardwick Collings (https://janehardwickecollings.com/) refers to this time as the time to share your autumn harvest (what you've learned in life), the time of healing ancestral maternal patterns. She describes an Indigenous saying that it's our time to weave dreams for the grandchildren. She puts forth the idea that insomnia and night sweats allow you to be awake at the time of your most powerful intuition, and we can look at that as an opportunity instead of a problem. And she urges us to look to nature to teach us how to navigate these challenges.

Only a few mammals actually experience menopause – narwals, pilot whales, orcas, belugas and humans. The menopausal members of these communities, the grandmas, are leaders of their packs – through their wisdom sharing, their descendants live longer and healthier.

This is called the grandmother hypothesis. It explains the existence of menopause in humans by identifying the adaptive value of extended kin networking. Originated by Kristen Hawkes, the grandmother hypothesis attempts to explain why menopause arose in human evolution, and how late-life infertility could actually provide an evolutionary advantage.

The hypothesis suggests that this is because of inherent risks associated with pregnancy, childbirth and postpartum, as well as the importance of parental (or grandparental) investment to the human species.

We can use this time to step into the initiation, embrace the gifts it brings us and allow it to empower us to bring our desires to fruition. This is what we are here at this moment in our lives to do … to step into our calling … to live our bliss … to bring our gifts and talents to the world.

Remember the commitment we made earlier: to create consistent rituals, start reducing menopause symptoms using natural methods and learn how to make this the most powerful phase of your life, while feeling sexy, vibrant and focused.

Let's do it together.

Menopause is Your Spiritual Initiation

FOLLOW YOUR BLISS

We can use this time of mid-life to step into the initiation, embrace the gifts it brings us and allow it to empower us to bring our desires into fruition. This is what we are here in this moment in our lives to do, to step into our calling, to live our bliss, to bring our gifts and talents to the world.

What is your bliss? What are you being called forth to do?

What will you bring to the world through this initiation of menopause?

Which quote about menopause as a spiritual initiation did you most identify with in this training? Why? How will you use that to step into your initiation?

VIBRANT MID-LIFE | Revolution

Chapter 3

Body, Mind, and Spirit: The Key to Radiant Wellness

We spoke earlier about how to reframe our cultural view of menopause … now we need tools to anchor that in.

Mindfulness is a very effective method of dealing with stress. And we know that stress contributes to most, if not all, of the issues we experience in midlife, including:

- Stress of all the cultural negativity around menopause.
- Stress from all the changes taking place externally.
- Stress from all the changes taking place internally.

Why is stress so intricately linked to menopausal symptoms? Here's the science:

Stress releases cortisol (cortisol is sometimes called the stress hormone), which leads to insulin resistance (where the cells don't respond to insulin), which leads to less energy (low glucose usage), which leads to elevated blood sugar, which leads to weight gain (from fat storage).

Stress =cortisol = insulin resistance = less energy = elevated blood sugar = weight gain

Inflammation from cortisol causes hormone receptors to shut down, which means there are more circulating hormones in the body. Cortisol also steals from progesterone production.

Symptoms from low progesterone include anxiety, PMS, low libido, dry vagina, irregular menstrual cycles, insomnia, infertility.

Cortisol = inflammation = hormone receptors shut down = more circulating hormones

Cortisol = low progesterone production

In terms of estrogen, stress leads to increased cortisol, which leads to the liver being unable to remove excess estrogen, which leads to increased estrogen or estrogen dominance. Symptoms of estrogen dominance can include rapid weight gain, fibroids, heavy periods, mood swings, insomnia, brain fog and low libido.

Cortisol = liver unable to remove excess estrogen = increased estrogen

In fact, even conventional medical sources are now confirming that stress plays a major part in all illness. The Centers for Disease Control and Prevention of the United States estimates that stress accounts for more than 75 percent of all doctor visits. And, according to Occupational Health and Safety news and the National Council on compensation of insurance, up to 90 percent of all visits to primary care physicians are for stress-related complaints.

Therefore, we know that stress, in a variety of ways, factors into our experience of this phase of our lives. And that also tells us that reducing and managing stress is vital to creating and maintaining optimal health – especially now, when so many things are shifting and changing during the perimenopausal, menopausal and postmenopausal years.

So, this is why stress reduction techniques and tools are so important for building the foundation of health during perimenopause and throughout the menopausal journey.

Research shows that mindfulness-based stress reduction (MBSR) helps people sleep better and feel less anxious, lowers cortisol levels and eases depression symptoms – again, all common issues during menopause. In fact, one study on MBSR from the University of Massachusetts Medical Center reported a reduction of up to 40 percent in the number of hot flashes experienced among the participants.

Thus, mindfulness can be a very effective tool in balancing out many of the root causes of the symptoms we might be experiencing during midlife. Beyond that, however, if what we are really desiring is to experience true wellness, the best years of our lives, living our dreams and passions, then mindfulness needs to not just be a tool that we pull out when we are feeling stressed, but a way of life.

Six Keys to Mindfulness

There are so many different mindfulness techniques that can be easily incorporated into your daily rituals and routines. Many mindfulness exercises can be categorized into these six main practices:

- Thoughts
- Presence
- Gratitude
- Breathwork
- Meditation
- Movement

The Power of Thought

One component of mindfulness is our thoughts. Dr. Christiane Northrup, author of *The Wisdom of Menopause, says,* "Every thought you think affects the membrane of each cell in your body immediately." Let me repeat that ...

> *"Every thought you think affects the membrane of each cell in your body immediately."*

That's a pretty powerful statement … and it means that our thoughts are pretty powerful. Our thoughts have a powerful effect on our bodies. So, it makes sense to choose our thoughts wisely. One simple mindfulness technique regarding your thoughts is this: Focus on thoughts and distractions that run through your mind, but don't judge them. For example, you might notice that a thought about work comes to your mind. Rather than worry about your thought, simply note the thought ("kids") and feeling ("worry") without dwelling on them. Then turn your attention back to the present moment. It is common for the mind to wander when a person begins to practice mindfulness. If that happens to you, it's OK. Keep trying. This is why mindfulness is called a practice – it takes practice to not judge your feelings and thoughts. It takes practice to stay in the present moment.

I encourage you to try it right now. What thoughts are running through your mind at this moment? What emotions do you feel? Just notice them, but don't judge them. Then turn your attention back to the present moment. Go ahead and try it now, then come back to the book.

How did it feel to do that exercise?

Was it easy for you?

Was it challenging to turn your attention back to the present moment?

I invite you to practice this exercise throughout your day and notice how much easier it gets with practice.

Here is one more technique you can practice to become more mindful of your thoughts:

If you struggle with anxiety or worry, imagine your mind as a blue sky and your thoughts as clouds. Now imagine those anxious or worrisome thoughts floating across your mind, almost the same as you would watch clouds float across the sky. Do not judge or resist your thoughts. Just let them pass by as you watch.

Again, I invite you to try it out right now. See your mind as an expanse of blue sky and imagine any worries you might have as clouds floating right on by without resistance or judgment. When you are done, come back to the book.

What did you notice about yourself when practicing this exercise?

Was it easy to allow the worry to float away?

Can you imagine how, with practice, this can reduce your anxiety on a daily basis?

A really effective practice for reducing the weight of stress and anxious thoughts in the first place is to do what I call a "media fast." Our news media outlets today fill our minds with sensationalized, intensely negative propaganda. A great thing to accompany your spring cleanse, or some of the new ways you're nourishing your body right now, is to set an intention to do a news fast. It could be a one-day fast, a one-week fast, a one-month fast or longer. This is a great way to set a new baseline for yourself by getting rid of external, extraneous stress in your life. Don't worry; you won't miss out on anything major happening in the world and you most likely will start to feel a huge weight lifted off your shoulders in the process.

Once you have started practicing some mindfulness techniques that allow you to release your attachment to your thoughts, and you've cleared a lot of negative thoughts out of your energetic space by doing a news fast, an effective next step to take is to practice the art of "reaching for a better feeling thought." I borrowed this phrase from Abraham-Hicks and it is one that really resonates for me.

Our feelings are a great barometer for how mindful we are with our thoughts. If we are having a negative feeling, it is a message to pay more attention to the thoughts we are thinking and perhaps practice one of the techniques I covered earlier.

Here is the next step: Whenever you are experiencing a negative feeling, reach for a better feeling thought. For example, if you are feeling anxious about a big presentation at work in the morning, after noticing this feeling, think of something that produces a more positive feeling in you. Perhaps you might think about the beautiful picture your child drew for you ... or look out the window and think about how lovely the tulips look in the front yard. Do this until the anxious feeling shifts into an emotion that feels better.

Being in the Present Moment

An important component of mindfulness is staying in the present moment, also known as practicing presence. But, what does being present really mean? Being present means focusing your complete attention on what is happening right now, in this moment – who you are speaking to, what you are feeling, the words you are using, using all your senses to ground you in the present moment.

Let's think about this linguistically. How is the word present defined?

One meaning is "a gift." So, you could say that allowing yourself to be present is a gift that you give yourself and those around you.

The present moment allows the stress of what happened yesterday and what may happen tomorrow to all fade away so we can enjoy the present (the gift) of the present (this moment) – interesting correlation, yes? We use the same word for the moment we are experiencing right now as we do for a gift. I think there is something really empowering in that.

Research shows that we are never happier within ourselves than when we are "present," no matter the activity. Harvard researcher Matt Killingsworth designed a mindfulness study of fifteen thousand individuals, which concluded that people who focused on their present moment experience were significantly happier than people whose minds wandered away from the moment. This is a big component of "mindfulness." Being present simply means we are paying attention to the activity at hand, even if it's mundane.

There are many ways we can practice being in the present moment. Many of them seem very simple, but don't let their simplicity fool you. These tools can be very powerful in helping you create true wellness in your life. I'd like to share a few of them with you now. The first is called the Object exercise:

Object Exercise

1. Pick up an object that you have lying around. Any mundane everyday object will do … a coffee cup or a pen, for example.
2. Hold it in your hands and allow your attention to be fully

absorbed by the object.

3. Observe it.
4. Don't assess it or think about it, or study it intellectually. Just observe it for what it is.
5. You'll feel a sense of heightened "nowness" during this exercise.
6. Conscious observation can really give you a feeling of "being awake."
7. Notice how your mind quickly releases thoughts of past or future, and how different it feels to be in the moment.

The next presence practice I'd like to share with you is called Using Your Senses:

Using Your Senses

1. Take a moment to consciously collect information about the world around you through your touch, your eyes, your ears, your smell and perhaps through your taste.
2. What can you see around you?
3. What can you hear around you?
4. What can you smell or feel?
5. Allow yourself a few moments to sit with the sensations you feel, as you focus on what you can observe with your physical senses.

Here's another similar but more intense presence exercise called the Task At Hand:

Task At Hand

1. Start by bringing your attention to the sensations in your body.
2. Breathe in through your nose, allowing the air downward into your lower belly. Let your abdomen expand fully.
3. Now breathe out through your mouth.
4. Notice the sensations of each inhalation and exhalation.
5. Proceed with the task at hand slowly and with full deliberation.
6. Engage your senses fully. Notice each sight, touch, and sound so that you savor every sensation.
7. When you notice that your mind has wandered from the task at hand, gently bring your attention back to the sensations of the moment.

These next two exercises can be challenging for many women. I urge you to be compassionate with yourself while you use these tools to get really present to this moment. These can be the most empowering of all when you allow yourself the time to nurture yourself in this way.

Three-Minute Mirror

1. I invite you to stand in front of a mirror – full length is best.
2. Look at yourself in the mirror for three minutes.
3. Practice your deep breathing and allowing all negative thoughts to pass by with no judgment.

The last presence exercise is called the I Love You Practice.

I Love You Practice

1. Take the last exercise one step further and continue to look at yourself in the mirror and say "I love you."
2. Repeat this as you look at every part of your body individually.

I'd like to ask you to pause right now and practice these last two techniques. Find a mirror and a quiet place where you can be alone for five minutes or so and practice the Three-Minute Mirror exercise and the I Love You Practice. Then come back to this book.

How did that feel for you?

Was it challenging?

Was it easy?

What did you feel in your body as you experienced these practices?

Can you see how using these tools on a daily basis to be present in the moment can shift things for you?

The Grace of Gratitude

Why gratitude? Thousands of years of literature talks about the benefits of cultivating gratefulness as a virtue and recent research has shown how the practice of gratitude can result in major health benefits.

For example, gratitude research suggests that feelings of thankfulness have tremendous positive value in helping people cope with daily problems like stress. There are also some very interesting findings linking optimism and gratitude to better immune function, better sleep and lower rates of depression, and according to a 2012 study, grateful people experience fewer aches and pains and they report feeling healthier in general than other people.

Now, you might be saying to yourself … I already have a gratitude practice … or … I'm already a grateful person … I don't really need this teaching. I know I have felt that way before when I am looking to expand my learning and yet it's important to have a beginner's mind whenever we are wanting to make changes in our life.

I'd like to share a story with you:

A Japanese Zen master received a university professor who came to inquire about Zen.

The Zen master served tea. He poured his visitor's cup full, and then kept on pouring. The professor watched the overflow until he no longer could restrain himself.

"It is overfull. No more will go in!"

"Like this cup," the Zen master said, "you are full of your own opinions and speculations.

How can I show you Zen unless you first empty your cup?"

Does this make sense to you? You may have already been exposed to many of the things we have talked about in this book, but there is always more to learn and there are always tools to go deeper. Here are a couple of other quotes about the beginner's mind:

"In the beginner's mind there are many possibilities; in the expert's there are few."

– Shunryu Suzuki-roshi

"When any real progress is made, we unlearn and learn anew what we thought we knew before."

– Henry David Thoreau

In terms of creating gratitude rituals, there are many simple but powerful ways to bring more gratitude into your daily life. For example:

Gratitude Journal

One way to create a gratitude ritual is by keeping a gratitude journal. This can be a special journal just for putting down in words what you are grateful for. It can be part of your morning ritual, your nighttime ritual, or both! You can write down one thing you are most grateful for, or you can make a list of everything you are thankful for in this particular moment. You get to choose how to weave using a gratitude journal into your life … and then see how many more things flow into your life that you are grateful for!

Morning/evening ritual of feeling your gratitude for the day

A related practice is feeling your gratitude for the day. This is a practice of embodiment. How does gratitude feel in your body? Take a few moments of breathwork and then bring to mind one specific thing that you are grateful for, such as your child, your pet, your home, the food on your plate or even just the fact that you woke up this morning. Ask yourself how it feels in your body? Where do you feel it in your body? Focus all your attention on that feeling, exactly where it is in your body and allow yourself to feel it fully.

Dr. Emoto's Work with Water Crystals

The next gratitude practice I want to share with you is based on Dr. Emoto's work with water crystals. Dr. Emoto studied how energy affects the crystalline structure of frozen water. His work is fascinating and I encourage you to learn more about it, if this interests you.

In a nutshell, what he discovered was that the energy of sound, words, and thoughts affects the structure of water. This resulted in either a chaotic, disorganized structure or highly organized, visually pleasing structure, depending on what the water was exposed to.

He found that the most beautiful water crystals were formed from being exposed to the energy, words, and sounds of gratitude and love. Since our bodies are composed mostly of water, this is highly significant to us as human beings.

Here's a way you can use this information to improve your health in a practical way. Place a piece of paper that says gratitude on it under or on your water container every day. Bring to mind something you are grateful for when you do this. Every time you drink that water, not only will the energy of gratitude fill you, but the note you have written will remind you to return to gratitude.

Say Thank You

A simple gratitude practice is to set an intention to say thank you to at least one person every day. Not only will this bring all the health benefits of a gratitude practice to you, but also those you choose to thank every day.

I'd like to leave you with one last thought. Have you heard the saying: What you focus on expands? When you focus on feeling grateful and expressing that gratitude, it attracts more things into your life to be grateful for.

Build Your Foundation with Breathwork

Another aspect of mindfulness is working with the breath. Focusing on your breath has the effect of putting you back into your body and being present in the moment. It can reduce stress, lessen anxiety, and relieve physical discomfort.

Andrew Weil, MD, (author of 8 Weeks to *Optimal Health*) states: "Conscious breathing is the most important thing we can do for our health, regardless of exercise and diet." Let me repeat that – "Conscious breathing is the most important thing we can do for our health, regardless of exercise and diet." That's a pretty remarkable statement and definitely something we all need to consider as we journey along the path to optimal health.

In direct relation to menopause, a 1992 study was conducted where physicians taught women who experience hot flashes to breathe slowly and diaphragmatically, which reduced the frequency and intensity of hot flashes by 50 percent!

One of the most effective breathing techniques there is, is deep belly breathing. This is also sometimes called diaphragmatic breathing. It sounds simple, and it is, but most of us don't practice this style of breathing on a regular basis.

Deep belly breathing consists of being conscious and intentional of your breath as you breathe deeply into the bottom of your abdominal cavity, filling it up from the bottom, up to the bottom of the lungs and then completely to the top of your lungs. Hold it for a few seconds and then exhale completely until you feel you have absolutely no more breath in you.

I find that a few deep belly breaths brings me back into the present moment and reduces all tension in my body immediately. Try it a few times now. Here are a few more breathing meditations that can be particularly effective for easing/reducing physical as well as mental and emotional symptoms very quickly.

- Breathing love and light into parts of our bodies where we feel pain of discomfort.
    - As you inhale, visualize love and light streaming in through your breath to those places in your body that are hurting, and as you exhale, visualize the pain leaving with your breath. Try it now.
- Breathing in love, peace or well-being, and then breathing out

anything less than that (I got this from spiritual coach Sharon Wilson and it's one of my favorites).

    - As you inhale, imagine that sense of well-being spreading throughout your entire body and as you exhale, imagine anything less than complete well-being being breathed out of your body. Try it now.

- Breath gratitude into all the billions of cells in the body that they know exactly what to do to stay healthy.
- As you inhale, visualize love and gratitude going directly into every single cell in your body and as you exhale, remind yourself that each one knows exactly what to do to be optimally healthy. Try it once now.

I want to mention that the effects are cumulative, so the more often you can practice breathing meditations on a regular basis, the more effective they become.

Here's an expanded view by creativity coach Robert McFadden on why the meditative practice of breathwork is so important to apply in daily life, especially when you need clarity and focus:

"Three elements in mindful meditation help in practicing how you focus your attention. The first is having a clear, concise point of focus. In the example above, the point of focus is the breath. The second element is awareness. That moment when you notice that your attention has shifted elsewhere. The third element is that little act of willpower to return your focus to your breath … Mindfulness breath meditation is a wonderful practice for developing awareness of your attention, exercising those little acts of willpower, and habituating setting priorities for focusing attention. It also provides a

marvelous model for how you can focus your attention in any situation, no matter where or when."

Is this making sense?

Can you see how powerful your breath can be?

And how it can help shift your health in so many positive ways?

There are a few more breathing exercises that I invite you to incorporate into your daily routine. They can be done anytime, especially if you are feeling stressed or holding tension in your body.

A good way to incorporate them into your daily routine is to start with the first one and then add the next exercise the following day/week and continue adding them incrementally until you are doing them all every day:

Breath Observation: Practice observing the breath for at least five minutes every day.

1. Sit in a comfortable position, back straight, eyes closed, loose clothing.
2. Focus attention on breathing, inhalation and exhalation, noting the points at which each phase blends into the other.
3. Continue for five minutes.

Beginning with Exhalation:

1. Focus attention on the breath without trying to influence it.

2. Experience exhalation as the beginning of each new breath cycle.
3. Continue for one minute.

Being Breathed:

1. Eyes closed, arms comfortable, focus on breath without influencing it.
2. Imagine with each inhalation the universe is blowing breath into you and with each exhalation withdrawing it. Let yourself feel the perception of each breath penetrating throughout your entire body.
3. Do ten cycles.

Relaxing Breath:

1. Tongue in yogic position – tip touching roof of mouth just behind teeth.
2. Exhale completely through mouth.
3. Close mouth and inhale through nose to count of four.
4. Hold for a count of seven.
5. Exhale through mouth for count of eight.
6. Continue for four cycles.

Stimulating Breath:

1. Sit in comfortable position, back straight, eyes closed, loose clothing, tongue in yogic position.
2. Breathe in and out rapidly through the nose, keeping mouth closed. Equal and short inhalation/exhalations.

3. Start with fifteen seconds. Increase daily by five seconds, until you get to full minute.

Incorporate the full breathing program into your day utilizing the following suggested schedule:

Integrated Breathing Program:

1. Morning: Stimulating, Relaxing, Breath Observation, Begin with Exhalation
2. Evening: Being Breathed, Relaxing

Remember, you don't need to practice all of these techniques, just try them out and choose a few that feel really good to you. Come back to this section as many times as you'd like to refresh your memory. Making one or more of these breathwork techniques part of your daily rituals is one of the keys to start reducing menopause symptoms using natural methods and making this the most powerful phase of your life, while feeling sexy, vibrant and focused.

Meditation Wisdom

In the goddess culture, Hestia is the Greek goddess of meditative wisdom in mature women. According to Jean Bakula, Hestia is the still point at the center of yourself. You yearn for your inner Hestia whenever you need some time and space for solitude. Hestia's symbolic fire warms and illuminates your mind and body, and gives you a sense of being at home in yourself.

> *"The time when your inner Hestia comes out is in the waning Moon, during your wise woman years. She is beyond the need or delusion that she needs someone or something outside herself in order to be complete. Hestia is perfectly at peace with herself just the way she is."*
>
> – Jean Bakula

One of the best ways to bring a healing practice of meditation into your daily routine is with a connection to nature. Exposure to nature makes you feel better! Not only emotionally – it contributes to your physical well-being, reducing blood pressure, heart rate, muscle tension, and the production of stress hormones. It may even reduce mortality, according to scientists. Research done in hospitals, offices, and schools has found that even a simple plant in a room can have a significant impact on stress and anxiety.

There is a strong body of research confirming that direct contact with nature increases mental health and psychological and spiritual development. Benefits include stress reduction, a sense of coherence and belonging, improved self-confidence and self-discipline, and a broader sense of community.

In fact, there is a Japanese therapy called shinrin-yoku, which translates to "forest therapy." Studies have shown markedly positive results for shinrin-yoku in decreasing stress responses and improving both physical and mental health markers.

One of the most common symptoms some women experience in midlife is poor memory and brain fog. According to emerging science, it appears that taking in the sights and sounds of nature is especially beneficial for our brains. Researchers at the University of Michigan found that performance on memory and attention tests improved by 20 percent after study subjects paused for a walk through an arboretum. Conversely, when these people were sent on a break to stroll down a busy street in town, no cognitive boost was detected.

If you have access to a green space and can take a nature walk every day, that is fantastic, but connecting with nature doesn't mean you need to clear your schedule for the weekend, drive to the mountains or the beach and meditate among the pines (although that sounds lovely). There are lots of simple ways to bring the healing power of nature into your home and daily life whether you live out in the country or in the middle of a bustling city. Here are just a few:

- Tend to a window herb garden in your kitchen for a few moments a day.
- Visit your favorite plant in your yard or balcony.
- Pet the cat lying on your lap.
- Create a display or altar in a special place in your house where you place natural objects that are particularly meaningful to you, like a stone or crystal, piece of driftwood or sprig of greenery or dried flower.

Spending time doing some of these things every day can help you reduce stress, improve brain function, sleep better and perhaps even extend your life! And these are all areas of health that are crucial to address during the perimenopausal, menopausal or postmenopausal years.

Audio meditations are a really popular way to bring meditation into your routine in a way that is easy and doesn't take up a lot of time. You can download and listen to them from a phone app or on your computer and you can listen to them upon waking in the morning, before bed at night, on a walk or at any time of the day when you need to find that place of stillness inside and focus on what's important to you at that moment.

I have created a meditation for you that you can find and listen to here: https://www.herbsofgracehealingarts.com/meditation. It is just an example of one way you can bring several of the components of mindfulness together. I encourage you to not only listen to it – in fact, you could download it and make it part of your daily mindfulness ritual – but I also invite you to create your own meditation and mindfulness practice that is unique to you. Something that you can look forward to every day!

I hope this helps you to see that meditation doesn't have to be difficult and it doesn't have to take a long time. You don't need to carve out an hour or even thirty minutes of your day to devote to meditating ... unless you want to. It can be a moment here or there throughout your day to tend to a plant in your yard, pet your cat or listen to soothing music. It can be a five- or ten-minute break in your daily work to listen to an audio meditation. These small daily habits make such a difference in our overall health and vitality. So, make the commitment to start creating an everyday meditation ritual to help you move forward along your Vibrant Midlife Goddess Path today!

Movement Meditations for Midlife

What do I mean by movement meditations? By this point we are fairly aware of what meditation is, but how many of us use movement as a meditation. The Free Dictionary defines meditation as a practice of concentrated focus on a sound, object, visualization, the breath, movement, or attention itself in order to increase awareness of the present moment, reduce stress, promote relaxation, and enhance personal and spiritual growth. I'd like to focus on the movement piece now because it's important for each of us to find what works best for us ... and I have found movement to be an incredibly effective form of meditation for me and my clients. And it could be for you too! Here are a couple more reasons:

Release and Integrate Energy

Moving our bodies helps us to release stuck energy. That is one of the reasons we feel so good after dancing for a few minutes or taking a brisk walk. In fact, it is commonly known that an animal's body will shake or tremble after a traumatic incident to help release the energy of the trauma, and therefore, the stress it may cause. And likewise, when we move our bodies intentionally, it helps us to release any blockages of energy that have built up and that allows us to take in new energy. When we are enhancing our personal or spiritual growth, as in the definition of meditation I mentioned earlier, movement can help us move out the old energy and clear the space for the new. Have you ever experienced this? Let me know in the chat if you have witnessed an animal do this or if you have done it yourself.

Embody the Learning and Healing

There is a hot term right now that explains the next reason I find movement so effective as a form of meditation ... and that is embodiment. What is embodiment? One of the definitions is this: To make part of a system or whole; incorporate. When we use movement as a meditation, it enables us to incorporate, or make part of our system, the energy of the meditation, or the healing we are receiving or the new concepts we are learning. Movement helps us to embody what we learn, to incorporate and integrate it fully into our entire being.

The type of movement doesn't matter as much as how often we move, how consistent we are with our movement and how intentional we are. In my practice, I focus on natural movement techniques. As a culture, we have become more and more sedentary and more focused on convenience. As a result, we don't move our bodies in the ways they were designed to move and we don't move nearly as often as we were made to. Natural movements such as sitting to standing, squatting, lifting with your legs, carrying things, walking the stairs, hiking, walking in nature and dancing have far-reaching effects when you do them consistently and with intention.

Many women in midlife feel like they need to work out harder and more often, go to the gym every day and increase the length and intensity of their exercise routines. Often, this leads to more stress on the body, which leads to ... you guessed it ... higher cortisol levels. We've already mentioned that high cortisol levels are the major underlying factor of many of the symptoms we can experience during the menopausal phase of life. Harder, more intense movement is not the answer! Gentle, weight-bearing, natural movement will not only help you relieve stress, but it can also be one of the keys to losing that midriff weight gain, sleeping well and increased energy and focus.

Personally, belly dance has been one of the most empowering forms of meditation in my life. For you, it might be yoga or working in your garden. Whatever it is, I encourage you to find the form of natural movement that helps you be present, moves your body in natural ways and eases your stress levels.

And, now that you've incorporated components of mindfulness, meditation, breathwork, presence, and gratitude into your daily and/or weekly rituals, I'm excited for you to experience how much more focused, relaxed and less stressed you are feeling. These rituals set the stage for all the useful and practical things we are going to be talking about next. So, let me know how you are integrating these practices into your life.

Body, Mind, and Spirit:
The Key to Radiant Wellness

DAILY PRACTICES

Mindfulness Thought Practices:
- Noticing Your Thoughts
- Blue Sky Exercise
- News Fast
- Reach for a Better Feeling Thought

Mindfulness Presence Practices:
- Object Exercise
- Using Your Senses
- 3 Minute Mirror
- I Love You Practice

Mindfulness Gratitude Practices:
- Gratitude Journal
- Feeling your Gratitude for the Day
- Infuse your Water with Gratitude
- Say Thank You

Breathwork Practices:
- Deep Belly or Diaphragmatic Breathing
- Breathing love and light into parts of our bodies where we feel pain or discomfort
- Breathing in love, peace or well-being, and then breathing out anything less than that
- Breath gratitude into all the billions of cells in the body
- Breath Observation
- Beginning With Exhalation
- Being Breathed
- Relaxing Breath
- Stimulating Breath

Meditation Practices:
- Nature
- Audio or Visualization
- Movement

Which Practices are you going to put into your daily ritual?
How do you feel after practicing them?

VIBRANT MID-LIFE | Revolution

Chapter 4

Nourish Your Symptoms Away

In this chapter, we'll explore what it means to be deeply nourished and why it's so critical to our health, especially at this juncture in our lives. I will also give you some practical and useful resources and tools you can put into practice every day to feel your best.

In the goddess culture, Annapurna Devi – the Hindu goddess of food and nourishment – is an avatar of Parvati, one of the numerous incarnations of Shakti, wife of Shiva. (Shakti is known as the representation of universal feminine energy.) Anna means "food" in Sanskrit and purna means "filled completely." Annapurna's statues are often found in Hindu kitchens for her blessings. It is believed in India and Nepal that when food is cooked with the spirit of holiness it is a form of alchemy. Annapurna blesses the food and converts it to amrita, which is the Sanskrit word for delicious and healthy food, which gives immortality.

As simple as it sounds, we really are what we eat! Our food choices affect every area of our health and life in general. For women specifically, when dealing with midlife changes, the first thing to address is food and how we nourish our bodies. In fact, there is a saying in holistic healing traditions, that no matter what health issue you are dealing with, "When in doubt, start with the gut."

We can trace this all the way back to Hippocrates who said:

"All disease begins in the gut." – Hippocrates

But what does this really mean in practical terms? From my perspective as a natural health-care practitioner, it means two things:

1. Everything we put into our bodies, every food, beverage, herb, supplement, and so on, is either affecting our body positively and giving it what it needs to support us, or it is affecting our body negatively and contributing to a state of dis-ease. And, as a result of that, only we have the choice, the responsibility to make those choices that will either support us or work against us. (By the way, this not only pertains to the physical things we put into our bodies, but also what we put into our mind, heart and spirit, which we already talked about in depth in the last chapter.)
2. We need to address the health of the gut before anything else. If our digestive tract cannot assimilate and metabolize what we are putting into it, those healthy choices we make in terms of food and herbs will not have the effect they have the potential to make. If we can't assimilate the nutrients we take in, our bodies can't make use of those nutrients to heal us and support our health. So, addressing and building optimal functioning of the gut is our

number one priority, especially when we are experiencing issues with our health.

What Does Poor Gut Health Look Like?

To give us a better understanding of what we can experience when we are not paying attention to nourishing our bodies with the foods we choose and not paying attention to our digestive health, here is a short list of just a few of the possible effects of poor gut health. Take notice if you are experiencing any of these effects of poor gut health:

- Autoimmune illnesses, such as celiac, Crohn's, ulcerative colitis, psoriasis, lupus and multiple sclerosis, to name a few
- Fatigue and low energy
- Food allergies
- GI issues, such as constipation, diarrhea, gas, bloating, etc.
- Mental health issues
- Skin irritations
- Sleep issues
- Unhealthy weight

I want to share a few studies with you that highlight a couple of these issues. In terms of mental health issues, studies suggest that digestive function may also affect certain cognitive functions, such as thinking skills and memory, as well as early Parkinson's disease. A 2015 Cell Journal study found that, although serotonin is well known as a brain neurotransmitter, approximately 90 percent of the body's serotonin is made in the digestive tract. A lack of this "peripheral" serotonin, which is cultivated by certain bacteria in the gut and affects mental health, has been linked to diseases like irritable bowel syndrome, leaky gut, cardiovascular disease, and osteoporosis. Serotonin, by the way, is also known as the happiness hormone. It helps stabilize your moods and affects your feelings of well-being, as well as your sleeping patterns and brain function. So, if you're experiencing any of these symptoms, low serotonin as a result of poor gut health could be a primary contributor.

In terms of unhealthy weight, there are two studies supporting this theory that are really interesting to me – one looking at mice, the other using humans – found that a family of bacteria known as Firmicutes (species of bacteria) was more plentiful in the obese (20 percent more), whereas another bacteria called Bacteroidetes (more bacteria) was almost 90 percent lower in obese subjects. Firmicutes appear to be more efficient at taking calories out of complex sugars and depositing those calories in fat (which makes you gain weight faster). In fact, when Firmicutes were transplanted into normal-weight mice, they gained twice as much weight while eating the same diet. In the human study, obese people who lost weight increased their Bacteroidetes, while the numbers of Firmicutes decreased. This indicates that one of the biggest factors in gut health is the balance between healthy and unhealthy bacteria colonies in the GI tract. We'll be talking more about this a bit later.

Why Nourishing is Better than Deprivation

Right now, I want to introduce to you the idea of deep nourishment. I invite you to consider the idea of deeply nourishing your body instead of dieting or depriving it of specific foods.

I believe we need to reassess the language we use around food.

What feelings do you associate with the words diet and dieting? Do they provoke positive feelings/energy or negative feelings/energy? If we want to nurture and nourish our bodies and set the stage for optimal levels of healing to occur, let's consider choosing words such as nourish, nurture, enrich and savor ... instead of diet, elimination, cutting out and depriving. Let's focus on additions to what you eat instead of subtraction; let's focus on enriching instead of depriving.

Another note on "diet" – I don't believe there is any one best diet. We are all individuals with unique needs that may change throughout our lifetime. We need to honor our diversity and cultivate an intuitive knowledge of what is best for us individually. We can do this through trial and error, observing our bodily responses, meditation, education, mentorship, and specifically through practices that strengthen our intuitive wisdom and connection between mind, body and spirit. Go back and review chapter 2 if you need inspiration with that.

One final note about eating and nourishing our physical bodies ... study after study has given us a clear picture regarding which foods are generally healthiest for most humans. I absolutely believe that this needs to be tailored to each individual's specific needs, which is why I love working one-to-one with women. But as a general rule of thumb, I love to quote Michael Pollan:

– *"Eat food. Not too much. Mostly plants."*

To expand on that:

- Eat whole, real, unprocessed foods.
- Eating as much of your foods in their raw, whole, unprocessed, organic state as possible is critical to healing and maintaining

health.

- If you are not able to obtain all your foods in an organic state, be sure at least to only consume animal foods that are organic. Pesticides, antibiotics and artificial growth hormones bioaccumulate in animal fats, so it is crucial to avoid them.

There are many other ways to nourish yourself than just nourishing your physical body. In the last chapter we discussed many techniques to nurture the mind, body and spirit connection … so I invite you to make an internal inquiry about what truly, deeply nourishes you. Some things that deeply nourish me are long warm mineral salt baths, spending time in nature, spending time with my children, and dancing!

Let's Get Practical

Next, we are going to be talking about very practical ways to bring deep nourishment and nurturing into our daily eating practices and rituals. So, how do we utilize our understanding of deep nourishment on a practical level?

I'm going to share with you many ways we can do that in this section. Some of these methods may seem very simple and some of them you may have heard before. However, don't write them off. They are incredibly effective steps to take on your healing journey. Sometimes the simplest things are the key to the greatest leaps in health.

- First up is hydration – drink pure water … and lots of it. Since our bodies are made up of more than 70 percent water, it is one of the most important aspects of our health. Did you know that experts believe that 90 percent of all headaches are caused by dehydration? A good way to keep your body hydrated is this: Whenever you feel the least bit thirsty or hungry – drink a glass of water first. If you need some more specific guidance, a good rule of thumb is to take your weight in pounds and divide it by two. Drink that much water in ounces per day. For example, if you weigh 150 pounds, you would want to drink 75 ounces of water per day.

- Also remember that city tap water contains many substances that are harmful to your body such as chlorine and fluoride. Make sure you either use a good filter or better yet, find a local source of spring water. Staying hydrated is imperative, so stay hydrated, but limit large amounts of liquids right before, during, and after meals. This can dilute your digestive juices, impairing the breakdown of your food. If you have a hard time drinking plain water, you can add slices of lemon, lime, cucumber or mint for flavor and extra nutrients.
- Lemon water – to piggyback on that last point, I want to talk specifically about lemon water. It does more than just hydrate. It promotes detoxification and peristalsis. What this means, in practical terms, is that a glass of lemon water first thing in the morning is a great way to get a jump start on your metabolism, help your body to detox and get your bowels moving. I have a great recipe for a way to rev up your lemon water I adapted from Dr. Lindsay Berkson that I will be sharing with you in the recipe section (pg. 176).
- Eat the rainbow – the constituents that make up the foods we eat play a part in the color of the food. Since it's crucial to consume a wide variety of nutrients every day, one simple way to make sure your body is getting everything it needs is to eat the rainbow. Make sure you eat natural, whole foods in as wide a variety of colors as you can.

- Eat at least two high-fiber foods each day. High fiber foods help feed good gut bacteria, assist in maintaining a healthy weight, lower the risk of obesity, diabetes, heart disease, and certain types of cancer. Examples of high fiber foods are whole grains; raw fruits with skins and dried fruits; raw or lightly cooked vegetables; nuts and seeds with skins; beans, peas, lentils; ground flaxseeds.
- Chew your food well. Remember our stomachs don't have teeth! The more work we do ahead of time, the better. This allows our digestive enzymes to do their jobs more efficiently and places less stress on the GI system. Try chewing each bite fifteen times; work up to thirty. See how you feel.
- Eat while relaxed and peaceful, taking time to enjoy your food and being aware of nurturing yourself. This could include creating a beautiful mealtime ritual to bring more intention to nourishing yourself.
- Eat until you are only three-quarters full. In many cultures we are often taught to clean our plate before getting up from the table. This not only encourages overeating, but ignores the signals your body is sending you. When you stop eating before you are feeling completely full, it allows the body to complete the process of digestion at a more easeful pace and we often find out when we do this that we are completely sated after all, eating less food.
- Avoid frozen and iced beverages and foods at mealtimes. The digestive process needs warmth and is hampered by excessive coldness.
- Avoid food triggers – earlier I talked about focusing on additions to your diet and not subtractions; however, if you know you have food triggers, sensitivities or allergies, it's obviously the wisest course of action to avoid them as much as possible.

- Intermittent fasting – this is a way of eating that has been talked about a lot recently. This refers to the timing of your meals. Making sure there are at least twelve hours between the last meal of the day and the next morning meal improves your metabolism, aids fat loss, creates positive psychological shifts, and eases brain fog and depression. You can experiment to see what the ideal fasting range is for you, but many women find twelve to sixteen hours between that last meal of the day and the first meal of the next day to be healthiest for them. If you have known thyroid issues or hypoglycemia, you'll want to be very cautious about implementing this practice.
- Bone broth – is nutrient-rich, easily digested and soothing to the digestive system.
    - A report published in the Journal of Clinical Gastroenterology found that gelatin effectively supports intestinal health and integrity.
    - If you are vegetarian, vegetable broth or miso is a wonderful alternative, although without the gelatin.
- Dark green leafy vegetables – I would be remiss if I didn't mention these wondrous delights. We have all heard many times how great these are for us ... and it's true. They are nutrient-rich, full of antioxidants and most are available all year round. The more of them you can get into your food plan, the better.
- Prebiotics – next up is prebiotics. By definition, prebiotics are a type of nondigestible fiber compound. The healthy bacteria in our gut love to feed on these foods, so getting more of them in your diet will help your good bacteria to flourish. Here's a list of prebiotics you can add to your diet:
    - acacia gum (or gum arabic)

    - raw chicory root
    - raw Jerusalem artichoke
    - raw dandelion greens
    - raw garlic
    - raw leeks
    - raw or cooked onions
    - raw jicama
    - raw asparagus
    - underripe bananas
    - raw honey
- Probiotics – last but not least, we have probiotics. We've talked about probiotics a bit already. This refers to the colonies of good bacteria in your gut that not only enable your digestive system to work efficiently, but studies have found that up to 80 percent of our immune system is in the gut. So in today's world, it is more important than ever to focus on the health of the gut and the probiotics that reside there. We've already spoken about the connection between gut health and cognitive function. Additionally, here are more examples of the connection between the gut and mood: In 2011, British scientists gave probiotics to both rats and human subjects. After a month, they noted a significant decrease in both the rats' anxiety-like symptoms and in the humans' levels of anger, distress, hostility, and depression. More recent research out of Oxford showed that supplements designed to boost the numbers of healthy gastrointestinal bacteria may improve anxiety levels by changing the way we process emotional information. The study participants were actually found to pay less attention to negative words and more attention to positive words after three weeks of supplementing. Examples of probiotic foods

that help establish and increase the good bacteria colonies in the gut are:

- beet kvass
- buttermilk
- dosa
- kefir (water and milk)
- kimchi
- kombucha
- lassi
- miso
- natto
- raw cheeses
- raw milk
- sauerkraut
- sourdough
- soy sauce
- tempeh
- yogurt

Why is Kombucha so Popular?

Speaking of kombucha … there have been a few recent studies on kombucha now that it has become so popular, and the verdict is that it can benefit many people:

- Kombucha has been shown to effectively heal gastric ulceration. Researchers believe the fermented tea protects the mucin content of the stomach. Its antioxidant activity also protects the lining of the gut. Kombucha also reduces gastric acid secretion that can damage the mucous membrane. In fact, kombucha has been found as effective in healing ulcers as prescription omeprazole (brand name Prilosec).

- Kombucha helps balance the metabolism. Animal studies show the tea may cause weight loss by encouraging calorie restriction.
- Research dating back to 1929 found kombucha can decrease blood sugar levels. More recent animal studies report that kombucha significantly reduces blood sugar levels in diabetic rats. Another study suggested kombucha may be considered a candidate for the treatment and prevention of diabetes.
- Kombucha protects against liver toxicity in animals from overdoses of acetaminophen (Tylenol).
- Kombucha contains strong antibacterials to combat infectious diseases such as diphtheria, dysentery influenza, paratyphoid fever, scarlet fever and typhoid. Its high total acidity makes it effective against Helicobacter pylori, Salmonella typhimurium, Staphylococcus aureus, and Bacillus cereus. It's been suggested that kombucha may be an effective alternative to synthetic antimicrobials that are becoming increasingly ineffective.

Falling in Love with Sauerkraut

Getting back to probiotics in general, you could certainly increase your healthy gut bacteria by taking purchased probiotic capsules. But a much tastier and more fun way is to make fermented foods. One of the easiest is sauerkraut. Traditionally fermented, homemade sauerkraut is not only a culinary delight but a big boost for your health!

- Most store-bought sauerkraut is not fermented in the traditional way and does not contain the billions of probiotics that the real stuff does. So, skip the store-bought and do it yourself!
- Making your own sauerkraut is simple and easy. I have included a tutorial for making your own sauerkraut below. Be sure to click the link and let me know how much fun you're having experimenting with the recipe! (pg. 175)
https://www.herbsofgracehealingarts.com/post/making-sauerkraut-how-to-make-your-own-sauerkraut-at-home

A small percentage of people cannot use probiotics until they heal other chronic conditions they have, such as SIBO (small intestinal bacterial overgrowth). So these suggestions are general recommendations that need to be personalized to your unique needs.

The last thing I want to mention here is nourishing infusions. These are a way to get high levels of nutrients into your body in an easy and effective way on a daily basis. I'm going to go into detail on this in the Unlock the Magic of Herbs chapter later in this book.

Start with the Gut to Relieve Menopausal Symptoms

Our next section is all about healthy eating for the relief of menopausal symptoms. We're going to be covering specific foods and nutrients that can reduce the specific symptoms you may be experiencing.

In previous chapters, we've spoken about stress relief techniques like mindfulness and meditation and how they can help reduce our symptoms as part of a regular routine. And we've spoken about how nourishing ourselves, especially our GI tract, is crucial at this point in our lives. Now, I want to get into some of the nuts and bolts of why that is. Understanding the endocrine system is a part of that. As we start getting into talking about the organs and hormonal glands here, I want to take a moment to explain what the gut/hormone connection is and why addressing digestion and gut issues is so important, especially during midlife.

The common denominator is stress. Simply put – digestive issues cause stress, and, here is a recap of how stress affects our hormones:

Cortisol: Stress releases cortisol, which leads to insulin resistance (where the cells don't respond to insulin), which leads to less energy (low glucose usage), which leads to elevated blood sugar, which leads to weight gain (from fat storage).

Inflammation from cortisol causes hormone receptors to shut down. Cortisol also steals from progesterone production.

Thyroid: Stress leads to increased cortisol, which leads to insulin resistance, which leads to decreased conversion of T4 (thyroid hormone thyroxine) to T3 (thyroid hormone triiodothyronine) (insulin is required for this), which leads an increased conversion of T4 to RT3 (reverse triiodothyronine) (which slows metabolism), which leads to the survival mechanism of fat storage.

Estrogen: Stress leads to increased cortisol, which leads to the liver being unable to remove excess estrogen, which leads to increased estrogen, which leads to increased thyroid binding globulin, which leads to a lower amount of thyroid hormone available to the body to regulate metabolism, which leads to lower estrogen (which regulates cholesterol and biodiversity).

The Hidden Benefits of Probiotics

One of the most effective and easiest ways to improve digestion and gut health is through the addition of probiotics to the diet. We've spoken about this at length, but there is another factor that I want to mention while we are discussing estrogen. There is a new understanding in how this relates directly to menopausal symptoms, which is this: The estrobolome is a subset of gut bacteria that are needed for estrogen metabolism. What this means is that some of the good bacteria help break down the estrogen in your body. When that good bacteria is not present in large enough numbers, you have more circulating estrogen in your body, which contributes to estrogen-dominant symptoms such as:

- Bloating (water retention)
- Breast swelling and tenderness
- Cold hands and feet (a symptom of thyroid dysfunction)
- Decreased sex drive
- Fatigue
- Fibrocystic breasts
- Foggy thinking, memory loss
- Hair loss
- Headaches (especially premenstrual)
- Irregular or otherwise abnormal menstrual periods
- Mood swings (most often irritability and depression)
- PMS

- Sluggish metabolism
- Thyroid dysfunction
- Trouble sleeping/insomnia
- Weight and/or fat gain (particularly around the abdomen and hips)

Estrogen dominance has also been linked to allergies, autoimmune disorders, breast cancer, increased blood clotting, infertility, uterine cancer, and ovarian cysts, and is also associated with acceleration of the aging process.

So once again, I am going to encourage you to consume probiotics and fermented foods, such as kefir, kombucha, sauerkraut, miso, and yogurt on a daily basis, even a bite at every meal.

We've spoken of the necessity of giving your liver a little extra TLC during this time in life. Kichari is a gentle, nurturing way to help nourish and fortify the liver – I have included a recipe here for you (pg 185). I suggest eating it for a week straight in spring and late fall for a much gentler way to nourish and support the liver, and throughout the rest of the year anytime you feel like you need a bit of gentle cleansing and want to give your liver a bit of love.

Supporting Your Adrenals with Adaptogens

Next, I want to share with you about adaptogens for adrenal support – adaptogens are medicinal foods that help the body adapt to stress. They work via the HPA axis, which stands for the hypothalamic/pituitary/adrenal pathway of the endocrine system, so they are vitally relevant to our discussion of hormone balance and midlife changes. We'll be talking more about herbal adaptogens in the Unlock the Magic of Herbs chapter. There are food adaptogens as well.

Here are a few of the most common that you can incorporate into your meals on a regular basis:

- chaga
- cordyceps
- goji berries
- huckleberries/wild blueberries
- nettle seeds
- reishi
- turmeric

Balancing Your Hormones with Phytoestrogens

Next up are phytoestrogens, which are plant hormones. They are weaker versions of our hormones and help the body to rebalance our fluctuating levels of hormones. They are safe, gentle and they don't have the side effects that pharmaceutical hormones have. They have the ability to lock on to estrogen receptors in the body and prevent harmful chemicals from disrupting hormonal signals. There are many plant foods that contain phytoestrogens; some of the best sources are: tofu, miso and flaxseeds. Including some of these foods every day can help to reduce symptoms and bring you back into balance.

Here is a more extensive list that you can come back to if you need a reminder:

- alfalfa sprouts
- aniseed
- apples
- barley
- beetroot
- brewer's yeast
- broad beans
- broccoli
- brown rice
- bulgur wheat
- cabbage
- carrots
- celery
- cherries
- chickpeas
- citrus
- clover
- corn
- couscous
- cucumbers
- dried apricots
- dried dates
- garlic
- green beans
- green split peas
- green squash

- hummus
- kidney beans
- legumes
- linseed
- mung bean sprouts
- nuts
- oats
- olive oil
- olives
- papaya
- peas
- plums
- poppy seeds
- potatoes
- pumpkin seeds
- red onions
- rhubarb
- rye
- sesame seeds
- soy
- squash
- sunflower seeds
- sweet peppers
- tofu
- tomatoes

Seed Cycling for Hormonal Balance

Another way to practice deep nourishment in midlife is seed cycling. Seed rotation is great for any woman experiencing symptoms of estrogen dominance or symptoms of low estrogen. Earlier, we went over the symptoms of estrogen dominance (pg 74).

However, low estrogen can also be a source of symptoms for women during the menopausal journey. Especially if we are experiencing a lot of stress in our lives, our hormone levels can drop quickly, causing quite a bit of discomfort and adding to our stress, which can cause a downward spiral. Here is a list of possible symptoms of low estrogen:

- an increase in urinary tract infections (UTIs) due to a thinning of the urethra
- breast tenderness
- depression
- fatigue
- headaches or accentuation of preexisting migraines
- hot flashes
- irregular or absent periods
- painful sex due to a lack of vaginal lubrication
- shifts in mood
- trouble concentrating

If you experience a number of these symptoms, you may want to consider adding seed cycling to your diet. Seed cycling helps balance your hormones, especially estrogen and progesterone. This is why it can reduce symptoms of both too much and too little estrogen.

The technique described here is based on a 28-day cycle. If your cycle is 28 days, then your seed rotation will be based on two 14-day cycles. Perimenopausal, menopausal and post-menopausal women, who don't have a regular cycle or any menstrual cycle at all, can start any day and rotate the seeds every two weeks.

Menstruating women have specific needs: From day 1 to day 14, we need more estrogen in order to build up our endometrium (uterine lining). This is called the follicular phase. Seeds such as flaxseed and pumpkin seeds, one tablespoon each per day, can naturally increase your estrogen levels.

From day 15 to day 28, or the second part of the cycle (also known as the luteal phase), the corpus luteum begins to release progesterone. This sex hormone will help thicken the uterine lining and prepare it for implantation. The high content of zinc in sesame seeds and vitamin E in sunflower seeds have been shown to stimulate progesterone production. By adding one tablespoon of sesame seeds and one tablespoon of sunflower seeds per day in the luteal phase, you can naturally support the body to produce more progesterone.

I give credit to Magdelena Wszelaki from Hormones Balance, from whom I learned this method.

In the last section, we covered foods that can nourish those of us who are specifically in the midlife phase of life, and now we're going to move on to the specific individual symptoms you may be experiencing and which exact foods can help reduce them. I'm going to start with weight. Because of hormonal imbalance and fluctuations, many women start to accumulate extra fat, especially around the waistline. Here are some specific food recommendations.

Finding and Maintaining YOUR Healthy Weight

Finding your own sense of body positivity is a personal and intuitive choice. Probiotics, again, are the number one place to start. Studies have shown very positive results for weight loss with only the introduction of probiotics in the diet and no other changes.

Warm lemon water first thing in the morning jump-starts the metabolism and peristalsis and helps the functioning of the liver; it is also very alkalinizing.

Speaking of water ... whenever you feel hungry, drink a glass of water and wait ten minutes before eating anything. Most of us have been conditioned to think that we are hungry when what our body is telling us is that we need hydration. If you drink a glass of water every time you feel hungry, you can retrain yourself to the real message your body is trying to send you.

Timing of meals – twelve to sixteen hours between last meal of day and next morning meal, improves your metabolism and energy levels, creates a short intermittent fasting period between your last meal and breakfast.

Eating protein at breakfast – this is especially important if you get munchies in the evening, which is a sign of hormone imbalance, specifically the hormone leptin, as well as too many carbs early in the day.

Increase healthy fats like coconut oil, organic grass-fed butter and olive and avocado oil (unhealthy fats are hydrogenated and trans fats, fried fats, canola, corn or cottonseed oils, in particular). Many people who are trying to lose weight are advised to go on a low-fat diet and they equate eating fat with gaining fat. In reality, fat doesn't create fat; sugar creates fat. When you deprive your body of healthy fats, it goes into survival mode and stores everything it can into the fat cells of the body. So in essence, a low-fat diet is creating more fat storage in your body. The critical factor is in knowing which fats are healthy and which are not.

In terms of sugars, modern cultures have created a food system in which the average person is eating one hundred times more sugar than we did only a century ago. This has created havoc in our bodies. The fad of sugar-free foods then developed, which added insult to injury by loading our bodies with toxic, artificial sweeteners, which cause a wide variety of illnesses, some chronic and devastating. And, none of this actually fosters health in any way. If you are experiencing uncomfortable weight gain during your menopausal journey, it's critical to decrease sugars in your diet, especially artificial sweeteners and processed white sugars. Healthier sugars, to use sparingly, are molasses, maple syrup and raw honey.

Keep a diet diary, or a food journal, so you can track your results and make correlations between the foods you eat and the symptoms you experience

And, finally, here's some great advice from herbalist Susun Weed:

"Give up dieting. Eat the widest variety of whole foods possible. Don't

make any foods absolutely forbidden. What you eat everyday has the most effect. The best way to stop worrying about weight gain is to eat ten or more servings of fruit and vegetables, three or more servings of whole grains, and a cup of yogurt daily. Eat a bowl of hot soup at the beginning of the meal. You will feel more sated and eat less. Cold soups and drinks do not have the same effect."

Reducing Hot Flashes

Hot flashes! ... Will they ever end?!

It is estimated that up to 80 percent of women will experience hot flashes during the menopausal years and up to 30 percent of them will experience hot flashes and or night sweats for a prolonged period of time. For some, that stretches between seven and eleven years!

The pattern of hot flashes is unique to each individual woman ... some experience only one or two throughout menopause and they're done. Some women have one or two every hour for years on end. Some are mildly inconvenient and some are debilitating. Scientists don't know for sure what causes hot flashes or the variations of them from one woman to the next, but the consensus is that it has to do with the fluctuations of estrogen in the body and how that affects the hypothalamus, which is the gland that regulates body temperature.

Again, we are wanting to nourish ourselves with foods that will help balance out and reduce those hormone fluctuations.

Many of the suggestions and recommendations from the first part of this chapter form the basis of your plan to address hormone fluctuations and will most likely be reducing your hot flashes already. However, there are a few that are more specific for hot flashes and night sweats. They include:

- All of the suggestions from the foods for healthy weight section, so make sure to go back and take a look to refresh your memory.
- Increasing foods rich in vitamins C & E is extremely helpful –
  - Vitamin C:
    - acerola cherries
    - amla
    - berries
    - broccoli
    - Brussels sprouts
    - cantaloupe
    - cauliflower
    - citrus
    - dandelion leaf
    - kiwi
    - peppers
    - pineapple
    - rose hip
    - spinach
    - tomatoes
    - violet leaf and flower
  - Vitamin E:
    - asparagus
    - avocado

    - broccoli
    - dark leafy greens
    - eggs
    - nuts
    - plant oils
    - salmon
    - seeds
    - squash
    - trout

- Include foods rich in phytoestrogens: *fermented soy, sprouted nuts and seeds, flaxseed, beans, split peas and chickpeas.* We spoke about phytoestrogenic foods earlier. Refer to pg 77 to see the full list again.
- And finally, avoiding hot spices, caffeine, sugar, simple carbs and alcohol is key for some women in reducing or eliminating hot flashes and night sweats.

Easing Symptoms of Insomnia

Many women experience insomnia at various times of their lives. As we enter perimenopause, those episodes of insomnia can worsen for some of us. And, since sleep is when our body rejuvenates, heals and repairs, it is critical to make sure we do everything we can to sleep well on a regular basis or we will be unable to take advantage of the body's innate ability to heal itself and symptoms will begin to appear. There are many factors that can result in sleep issues for women in midlife and it is generally necessary to take an individualized approach. However, there are many common causes that we can address.

One of them is experiencing hot flashes or night sweats that keep you from falling asleep, or wake you up once you do. If this is you, make sure to go back to the hot flashes section of this chapter and take note of the suggestions there.

Another is depression, anxiety or mood swings. We will be addressing this in the next section, so make sure to pay special attention to those suggestions.

All of the suggestions from the foods for healthy weight section are appropriate for improving sleep also, particularly the timing of meals and the morning protein.

- The recommendations for increasing foods rich in vitamins B, C, D and E also are critical here:
    - Vitamin B:
        - avocados
        - brown rice
        - buckwheat
        - dark leafy greens
        - egg yolks
        - fish
        - nuts and seeds
        - organ meats
        - polenta
        - sweet potatoes
        - whey

- Vitamin C: see list on pg 84.
- Vitamin D, which is also considered a hormone, can be very helpful for relieving insomnia : The journal *Medical Hypothesis* published a research study that followed 1,500 patients over a two-year period. A consistent level of vitamin D3 was maintained in their blood over many months. This produced normal sleep patterns in most of the participants, regardless of their type of sleep disorder. Foods rich in vitamin D include:
    - butter
    - cheese
    - cod liver oil
    - egg yolk
    - fish
    - mushrooms
    - yogurt
- Increasing foods rich in vitamin E has also been found to help reduce insomnia. Vitamin E: see list on pg 84
- Increasing foods rich in the minerals potassium, iodine, calcium, magnesium and iron can help reduce insomnia and the fatigue that results from it:
    - Potassium:
        - cabbage
        - celery
        - seaweed
    - Iodine:
        - leafy greens grown in gardens fertilized with

seaweed

    - mushrooms
    - seaweed
    - unrefined sea salt

- Iron:
    - chocolate
    - liver
    - red meat
    - seaweed
- Calcium:
    - beans
    - dark leafy greens
    - legumes
    - raw nuts and seeds
    - tempeh
- Magnesium:
    - almonds
    - brazil nuts
    - brown rice
    - cashews
    - chocolate
    - kidney beans
    - pecans, rye
    - swiss chard
    - soybeans

- Making sure your last meal of the day is several hours before you go to bed and avoiding consuming caffeine, alcohol, spicy foods, and high-fat foods late at night are helpful as well.

Managing Mood Swings

Have you suddenly begun crying during sad commercials? Snapping at your teenagers when you used to be calm? Had a meltdown during a staff meeting, seemingly out of nowhere? The wildly fluctuating hormones of menopause may be to blame. When we think of the hormone production that starts shifting during midlife, we generally think only about estrogen and progesterone, but there are many other hormones involved. Estrogen helps to regulate several hormones, which have mood-boosting properties. These include:

- dopamine
- norepinephrine
- serotonin

Studies show that more than 50 percent of women experience mood swings during the menopausal years. These can include:

- Aggressiveness
- Anxiety
- Depression
- Excessive joy
- Feelings of helplessness, worthlessness, and/or hopelessness
- Irritability
- Sadness

So, what's a woman to do? Start with what she's eating, of course! All of the suggestions from the foods for healthy weight section apply to moods as well. Additionally, poor sleep contributes greatly to mood, so take a look at the foods for sleep section again too. Specifically, increasing foods rich in the B vitamins and vitamin C, will help address these symptoms.

- Vitamin B: see list on pg 86
- Vitamin C: see list on pg 84.
- Increasing foods rich in magnesium is also important – see list on pg 89.

If depression is a specific issue – focus on adding bitter foods to your eating rituals, as well as flaxseeds and avoid alcohol and caffeine. Here is a list of bitter foods that can help ease depression:

- apple cider vinegar
- artichoke
- arugula
- bitter melon
- broccoli rabe
- Brussels sprouts
- coffee
- cranberries
- dandelion greens
- dark chocolate
- eggplant
- endive
- grapefruit
- kale

- saffron
- sesame seeds

Banishing Brain Fog

About 60 percent of women over forty report "brain fog." Some clinical studies support this. Brain fog can include symptoms such as:

- Communication issues
- Forgetfulness
- Getting things mixed up
- Missing important details
- More time needed to process information
- Reduced mental clarity
- Trouble making decisions

If you experience any of these symptoms, take heart in the knowledge that you are not alone and studies confirm that during the menopausal years, while the hormones are fluctuating, especially due to the drop in estrogen, brain fog can be a temporary experience, but, fortunately, as those fluctuations diminish during post-menopause, these symptoms tend to disappear as the brain compensates. Research shows that one of the ways this happens is through the body increasing blood flow to the brain. To help balance and stabilize these fluctuations, there are many things we can do.

First, we can go back to the addition of phytoestrogens to the diet. You can review that list on pg. 77.

In addition, all of the suggestions apply from the healthy weight section, so please go back and take a look at the suggestions provided there.

And since brain function is closely linked to the quality of sleep you are experiencing and the quality of sleep you have may be linked to your experiences of hot flashes and night sweats, the suggestions in those sections are highly relevant as well. Omega-3 essential fatty acids are vital nutrients for healthy brain function that can fight inflammation and menopause-related mental decline. So including these in your daily intake can help greatly.

- Foods rich in omega-3 fatty acids include:
    - chia seeds
    - cod liver oil
    - fish such as mackerel, salmon, and herring
    - flaxseed
    - oysters
    - walnuts
- Good fats, in general, are critical for brain growth and health. Good fats include not only the essential fatty acids like the omega-3s we just mentioned but also:
    - avocado
    - coconut oil
    - grass-fed organic butter
    - nuts
    - olive oil
    - wild-caught salmon

- Vitamin E is a vital component of brain health because of its strong antioxidant properties, which protect brain cells against damage from free radicals that occur naturally in the body and come from outside pollutants:
    - Vitamin E: see list on pg 84.
- Vitamin B is also critical to brain health:
    - Vitamin B: see list on pg 86.
- Vitamin C is another component of keeping the brain optimally healthy.
    - Vitamin C: see list on pg 84.
- Antioxidants such as lutein, zeaxanthin and anthocyanins are powerful brain boosters as well. Foods rich in these antioxidants include:
    - avocado
    - blackberries
    - blueberries
    - collard greens
    - kale
    - mustard greens
    - raspberries
    - spinach
    - strawberries
- And finally, I want to reiterate the importance of probiotics. Earlier, we learned how our digestive health is directly related to our cognitive health. And we also learned that a really potent way to increase the level of your gut health is through probiotics. Examples of probiotic foods that help establish and increase the

good bacteria colonies in the gut can be found on pg 69.

A Word About Inflammation

This was a powerful chapter, so congratulations on all you've learned about how to nourish yourself deeply to create lasting, vibrant health and reduce your menopausal symptoms naturally. Before moving on to our next chapter, there are a couple of things I want to mention when it comes to deeply nourishing ourselves ... and one of them is regarding inflammation.

I want to address the issue of inflammation for two reasons – firstly, many of my clients with menopausal symptoms are also experiencing inflammation. And secondly, I want you to see how this all ties together. Chronic inflammation may very well be an underlying factor with all of the specific symptoms we just covered and is a crucial factor in almost all disease (as research is now pointing to). So it needs to be addressed.

Everything that we have discussed in this entire chapter applies to reducing inflammation as well as the specific symptoms we talked about. Some of the root causes of inflammation are related to diet, sleep, stress and immune function – all things we talked about being some of the most common issues women experience during midlife. It is all tied together with the inflammatory responses of the body:

1. Bringing your gut bacteria into balance through probiotics dramatically increases immunity, cognition and positive mood and lessens chronic inflammation.
2. Using adaptogenic foods helps us to better deal with stress, lessening the inflammation from the stress response.

3. Using the nourishing principles we have discussed throughout this module helps us sleep better, allows our bodies the restful time they need to heal properly and results in reduced excess inflammation.

Keep it Simple, Sister!

I want to emphasize that there is no one best diet for everyone and not every suggestion in this chapter will be useful for every woman. We are all unique individuals, our bodies are unique and we each need to tap into our inner wisdom to know what is right for us. Working with a knowledgeable mentor can be critical to customizing your eating plan for optimal results.

And it's easy to get overwhelmed with so many food choices and so many recommended options. Just take things one step at a time. Eating healthy and using food as medicine doesn't have to be difficult. In fact, it can be incredibly simple. Let me tell you about my client Sheryl, who changed one thing in her diet and her issues were resolved from that one simple change.

Sheryl came to me because she had been suffering from lifelong eczema. The patches of rough, red, irritated skin caused her embarrassment, low self-confidence and anxiety anytime her skin was exposed. As a performer, this hindered her ability to show up on stage and perform at her highest level. After a thorough intake, we decided to start with making just one change at a time in her diet. The first thing she agreed to do was to stop drinking diet soda and replace it with plain water. A few weeks later, her eczema had completely disappeared!

That one thing changed everything for her! It's not always that simple, but using food as medicine and deep nourishment is often easier than people think.

Getting Out of Your Own Way

The next thing I want to address is that I am aware that you can learn nutrition in a lot of other places, but one thing you can't learn anywhere else is ... what is the thing inside of you that is keeping you stuck? Only you know that ...

What's keeping you stuck in your unhealthy eating habits?

What are you getting out of it?

Whenever we have a pattern that we want to change, but we have not been able to (such as experiencing excess weight or pain), there is always something that we are getting out of staying there. Perhaps it is fear of the unknown. We know we can live with the issue we have been dealing with ... but we don't know what's going to happen when it's gone and the primitive part of the brain wants to keep us safe by staying with what we know. Is safety what you are getting out of staying stuck?

Or perhaps it is protection ... Many women carry extra weight as protection – protection from being seen as who we really are, protection from unwanted advances, protection from doing what we need to do to become who we were really meant to be in this life.

Is protection what you are getting out of staying stuck?

My question for you is ... Can you release that?

Can you accept the possibility that you will be safe and protected without it?

If you feel ready to release what's keeping you stuck, I encourage you to seek support to help you do that in a way that is nurturing and will help you move forward. It's so important to address this before you go any further.

A Final Word of Encouragement

This was a really big chapter packed with lots of information and I know it's easy to feel overwhelmed. That's why we chunk it down into bite-sized sections. But I want to remind you that when it feels hard, that's OK. If this was easy, you wouldn't need this book. If this was easy, nobody would need support. It's OK for things to feel hard … that's why I do this work and why I'm here to support you.

One last thing I want to share with you – maybe the most important thing. *You are as powerful as you allow yourself to be.* I say this with absolute love and because I have been there.When you complain about things being too hard, too overwhelming, make excuses for why you can't do something, achieve something, and so on, you are giving your power away. *You are as powerful as you allow yourself to be.* I'm taking a stand for you today to stop giving your power away. Take your power back and let's do this together!

Nourish Your Symptoms Away

FOODS FOR MID-LIFE

Foods for Mood

- Foods rich in Vitamin B and C
- Foods rich in Magnesium
- Adding bitter foods is depression is a factor for you specifically

Foods for Sleep

- Foods rich in Vitamin B, C, D & E
- Foods rich in the minerals: Magnesium, Potassium, Iodine, Iron and Calcium
- Avoiding hot spices, caffeine, alcohol, high fat foods and eating at night

Foods for Flashes

- Foods rich in Vitamin C
- Foods rich in Vitamin E
- Foods rich in Phytoestrogens
- Avoiding hot spices, caffeine, sugar, simple carbs and alcohol

Foods for Healthy Weight

- Probiotics
- Lemon Water
- Drinking water when you feel hungry
- Timing of meals
- Eating Protein at breakfast
- Increasing healthy fats
- Decreasing sugars

Foods for Brain

- Foods rich in phytoestrogens
- Foods rich in Vitamin B, C and E
- Foods rich in Omega 3's and good fats
- Foods rich in the antioxidants - lutein, zeaxanthin and anthocyanin

Which of the foods from this chapter will you incorporate into your own daily ritual to create optimal nutrient uptake and vibrant health?

VIBRANT MID-LIFE | Revolution

Chapter 5

The Secrets of Energy Medicine

In this chapter, we will be learning that everything is energy and we will be addressing menopausal symptoms using vibrational remedies. You will come away with simple tools and techniques you can use to support your health, reduce symptoms and an understanding of how to use energetic remedies. But first I want to acknowledge that we are at the halfway mark! Yay! We have covered so much already and you have learned many effective tools and techniques to help you bring vibrant energy and wellness into your life. It's important to acknowledge our accomplishments and give gratitude for the progress we've made. I want to congratulate you on the healthier choices you have incorporated into your life.

Vibrational medicine is based on the premise that everything is energy. When I was young, I was taught in school that everything in the universe is made up of one of two things: either matter or energy. Now, quantum physics has scientifically shown us that all matter is actually energy, and that everything in the universe is made up of energy. All those energies just vibrate at different frequencies, making them appear either more or less dense to us, and therefore more or less solid. That means that our bodies also are made up of energetic systems. If that is true, then it follows that our bodies are affected by energy as well.

And, speaking of the concept that everything is energy – in the goddess culture, the goddess Shakti embodies the active feminine energy. Shakti is the subtle energy that means "power" or "empowerment," the primordial cosmic energy, and represents the dynamic forces that are thought to move through the entire universe in Hinduism. In a less overarching sense, shakti is the energy within everything.

Going back to a more scientific perspective, Dr. Richard Gerber, author of *Vibrational Medicine*, says, "Through his famous equation, E=mc2, Albert Einstein proved to scientists that energy and matter are dual expressions of the same universal substance. That universal substance is a primal energy or vibration of which we are all composed. Therefore, attempting to heal the body through the manipulation of this basic vibrational or energetic level of substance can be thought of as vibrational medicine."

He goes on to say, "Vibrational medicine attempts to heal illness and transform human consciousness by working with the energetic patterns that guide the physical expression of life."

Ancient societies have always acknowledged the importance of the energy pathways in the body and that healing takes place through clearing and unblocking these pathways. For example, in Traditional

Chinese Medicine this universal life-force energy is called chi, in the Hawaiian healing practice of Huna it is called mana and in the Indian subcontinent practice of Ayurveda it is called prana. The Chinese describe the energy paths as meridians and in Ayurveda, they describe the energy centers as chakras. Acupuncture, acupressure and reflexology, as well as many other healing modalities, all utilize knowledge of these energetic systems to achieve health and healing.

Albert Szent-Gyorgyi, Nobel laureate in medicine, states, "*In every culture and in every medical tradition before ours, healing was accomplished by moving energy.*"

In the following sections making up Chapter 5, I'm going to talk about three different types of vibrational health modalities and how they can help us through midlife and any challenges we experience along the way. These three vibrational medicine methods are:

- Flower essences
- Homeopathic remedies
- Energy medicine

Flower Essences

What are flower essences? Flower essences are gentle but powerful remedies made from the flowers of various plants. The use of flower essences is an energetic form of healing that can address mental and emotional, as well as physical, symptoms, although they are prescribed mainly for mental or emotional states.

Dr. Edward Bach created this system of energetic medicine in the 1930s, through his work with homeopathy, but, utilizing only the flowers of nontoxic plants and using only solar infusion of the flower's energies into pure spring water. He was an extremely sensitive healer and chose his original thirty-eight flower remedies through intuition and experimentation on himself and his students. He sought to create a gentle, nontoxic, but profoundly effective modality of healing that was built on the knowledge that the body is capable of curing itself. And so, the Bach Flower Remedies were born.

Since then, there have been many other organizations and companies that have discovered uses for hundreds more than the original thirty-eight remedies used in the Bach system. The American company FES (Flower Essence Society) and the Australian company Australian Bush Flower Essences, for example, carry hundreds of essences. There is also a wonderful Scottish company, The Living Tree, that creates flower essences only from orchids – very exquisite!

The Bach Flower Remedies are usually found at most health food stores. The others are available online. Flower essences are very easy to take, are incredibly safe, have no contraindications and act on a profoundly deep level. Generally, the dosage is two drops on or under the tongue several times a day, although in intense situations, they can be taken every five minutes.

Research supports the use of flower essences in treating disease on the emotional and physical level. A 2009 study by Marisol Oliva i Segura found that over 87 percent of the participants experienced an improvement in their emotional outlook and concluded that Bach Flower therapy appears to be a good alternative to psychopharmaceuticals.

Another interesting study was done in the area of pain management, which is often a very challenging condition to address. In this study by Judy Howard, 46 percent of the participants felt treatment had relieved their pain and about 88 percent of all subjects reported an improvement in their emotional outlook.

I have been using flower essences for more than twenty years now, and what I can tell you is that, if you are used to the effects of pharmaceuticals, meaning that you want to take a pill and perhaps feel a pretty immediate effect, and worry about the side effects later … that's generally not what you are going to get with energetic remedies. Flower essences, homeopathy, and energy medicine all work on a much deeper level to bring the body back into balance and support it to heal itself. So, what that might look like is a gradual shift in your feelings, thoughts and physical perceptions, perhaps better sleep, less anxiety and then perhaps the realization that that issue that had been nagging you for several months has disappeared, or that pain that you had gotten used to feeling is no longer there. The shifts can be very subtle but are often extremely profound.

In terms of menopause, there are several flower essences that can be helpful for a variety of issues.

- Walnut – This flower essence can help a woman adjust to the hormonal fluctuations and emotional changes that can occur during perimenopause and menopause. Many women also find it helpful for hot flashes. It is a remedy that is useful during times of change and can help us to adjust to the shifts that are taking place.
- Cherry Plum – This remedy can help restore calm and a sense

of control when overwhelmed by hot flashes, intense emotions or irrational explosiveness. Cherry Plum is for the woman who fears that she is going to lose control of herself.

- Olive – This flower essence can restore your energy when you've suffering from sleepless nights. It can help when there are feelings of complete exhaustion, where there are no reserves of energy left, when exhaustion occurs at the physical, emotional, and psychological levels so that the smallest task becomes an insurmountable obstruction. Olive can bring peace, restoration and balance.
- Scleranthus – This remedy can bring back balance to the woman whose swinging moods find her feeling joyful one moment and crying in despair or yelling in frustration the next. It is also for those who can't make up their minds and thus never commit to any clear decisions. When a woman is clearly out of balance – but is constantly seeking to find that balance and clarity of mind – Scleranthus can help her to make decisions quickly and with intuitive confidence.
- Crab Apple – This essence is also known as the cleansing remedy. Oftentimes, as a woman's body changes during and after menopause, she can become disillusioned with herself and have a hard time identifying with the beauty in the changing look and feel of her physicality. Crab Apple can help her to feel better about herself and her body. It can help nourish a woman's self-image and restore her confidence.

Homeopathy

What is homeopathy? There are many misunderstandings where homeopathy is concerned and many people think homeopathy just means "home remedies." Actually, homeopathy is an entire natural healing modality. It is beyond the scope of this book to undertake a full explanation of this healing modality, but suffice it to say that it has a proven track record of safety and efficacy, not only in terms of time (over 250 years' worth) but also meticulous record keeping and scientific research.

Homeopathy is a very safe, effective and gentle healing art that was founded in the late 1700s by a physician named Samuel Hahnemann in Germany and is practiced by close to five hundred million people around the world today. The practice of homeopathy is based mainly on three fundamental principles:

1. The law of similars
2. The infinitesimal dose
3. The treatment of the whole person

Let's take these one by one. The first fundamental principle of homeopathy is based on the law of similars, the principle of "like cures like." Hahnemann called this the similimum. This has also been stated as *similia similibus curentur* – let like be cured by like. This concept has been acknowledged since the times of the ancient philosophers and physicians. Hippocrates, Galen, and Paracelsus have all touched on the philosophy of the law of similars.

This law refers to the concept that a disease can only be cured by a remedy that produces the same or similar symptoms, when given to healthy people, that the disease produces in those who are afflicted with it. So, for example, a condition like hay fever, which produces uncomfortable, watery eyes and runny nose would be treated with Allium cepa (a remedy made from the onion plant) because onions can produce the same symptoms in a healthy person.

The second principle of homeopathy is that of the infinitesimal dose. One of Hahnemann's driving forces behind his search for a better system of medicine was his disdain for the medical treatments of the time. The administration of massive doses of poisonous medicines, common at the time, led him to state in his book, the *Organon*, "The highest ideal of therapy is to restore health rapidly, gently, permanently; to remove and destroy the whole disease in the shortest, surest, least harmful way, according to clearly comprehensible principles."

He designed his original provings to gradually reduce the dose of the remedy to determine the smallest dose that would still remain therapeutically effective. By coincidence, what he found was that not only are infinitesimally small doses even more therapeutically effective, but they are also completely free from the side effects that may be present in larger doses.

The last principle is the treatment of the whole person. Homeopathy is a very individualized modality of medicine. It aims to treat the whole person, to bring about a rebalancing of the vital force, and a complete disappearance of all symptoms, or in other words, a total cure.

In homeopathy, the remedy is matched to the individual, as well as to the symptoms, so people who have the same symptoms may receive different remedies. The entire makeup of the patient –their constitution – is taken into consideration when choosing a homeopathic remedy. Hahnemann says in the *Organon:* "In bringing about a cure the physician should consider: the evident physical constitution of the patient (especially in chronic affections), his affective and intellectual character, his activities, his way of life, his habits, his social position, his family relationships, his age, his sexual life, etc." The remedy is matched in every way to the patient – physically, mentally, emotionally, spiritually, according to lifestyle, environment and family medical history. Determining whether a person is anxious, overweight, straightforward and light-haired, or confident, thin, artistic and dark-haired can make all the difference in prescribing the correct remedy for that particular person. This shows that homeopathy is indeed a "wholistic" form of treatment and it is, in fact, the third principle of homeopathy – to treat the patient as a unique individual and not just a set of symptoms, or the bearer of a disease.

Throughout the last century, homeopathy has been attacked by mainstream media and conventional medical organizations over and over. However, there is substantial empirical and scientific data to support its efficacy. In fact, in 2011 the government of Switzerland released the most comprehensive governmental report ever written on homeopathy and affirmed that homeopathic treatment is effective, cost-effective and safe. Additionally, the report concluded that homeopathic treatment should be reimbursed by their country's national health-care system.

There are many ways homeopathy can support a woman throughout her life, including through the changes occurring in midlife. One of the most effective ways is to work with a homeopathic practitioner and find your constitutional remedy. That is the remedy that fits your personality and can be taken for most any symptom because it helps your body to rebalance itself and activate its own innate healing abilities.

However, there are also several specific remedies that have proven helpful in particular situations experienced often during menopause.

Homeopathy for Hot Flashes

For hot flashes, one of the following remedies might fit your symptoms:

- Lachesis: If your flashes emanate from the top of your head, are worse just before sleep and immediately on waking and are accompanied by sweating, headaches, or easily irritated skin.
- Sepia: If your flashes make you feel weak, nauseated, exhausted, and depressed.
- Pulsatilla: If you flash less outdoors, but your flashes are often followed by intense chills and emotional uproar.
- Valeriana: If your face flushes strongly during the flash, and you have intense sweating and sleeplessness.
- Ferrum metallicum: If your flashes are sudden; your general health is good but ordinary activities bring exhaustion.
- Sulfuricum acidum: If your flashes include profuse sweating and trembling, are worse in evenings or with exercise.
- Sanguinaria: If your cheeks are red and burning, feet and hands hot.
- Belladonna: If the flash centers on your face, which burns and turns bright red; you are restless, agitated and have palpitations.

Easing Insomnia with Homeopathy

For insomnia, you might consider:

- Nux vomica: If you go to sleep late because of a feeling of thoughts crowding in. You wake at 3 a.m. and lie awake until daybreak, when you fall into a dull sleep full of dreams, from which it is hard to rouse. If you wake up late, feeling tired. Or if you experience sleeplessness and excitement after overwork or over-stimulation.
- Coffea: If you experience complete sleeplessness and are constantly moving and excited. You sleep until 3 a.m., after which you are only able to doze. Then you wake up with a start and feel excited. Your sleep is disturbed by dreams. Or you experience sleeplessness because of mental activity; have a flow of ideas, accompanied by nervous excitability.
- Belladonna: There is pulsation of the blood vessels, and you may hear this so loudly when trying to sleep as to be kept awake by it. You experience comatose sleep at night, with frequent waking and convulsive movements. Sleep may be accompanied by moaning and tossing about. There may be nocturnal sleeplessness, sometimes with the desire to sleep and useless efforts to go to sleep, mostly because of feelings of great anguish or agitation.
- Chamomilla: If you experience nocturnal sleeplessness, with attacks of anguish, visions and illusions involving sight and hearing. On sleeping, you start with fright, cry out, toss about, are tearful, talk, rave, groan, snore and constantly separate the thighs. There are fantastic, lively, quarrelsome and vexatious dreams, with a morose and sullen aspect.

- Aconite: There are nightmares and anxious dreams. You experiences sleeplessness, and are restless and toss about. You start up in sleep, have long dreams, with feelings of anxiety centered on the chest. If you experience drowsiness, with anxious thoughts and rapid respiration. This is especially associated with fear of dying and sleeplessness because of anxiety, constant agitation and tossing about.
- Arsenicum: If you feel disturbed, anxious, restless, agitated and toss and turn in bed. You must have your head raised by pillows. If you have suffocating fits during sleep. You sleep with your hands over your head. Your dreams are full of care and fear. You are usually worse at or after midnight.
- Gelsemium: If you have sleeplessness from anticipatory anxiety. You have a dull, drowsy mind – hard to think yet difficult to go to sleep. You experience insomnia from exhaustion, but it's hard to get fully asleep.
- Phosphorus: Used for sleeplessness in older people. You go to sleep late and awaken feeling weak. If you experience short naps with frequent waking. You have vivid dreams of fire or of hemorrhage. You may have lascivious dreams. You have anxious, distressing dreams that are frightful and horrible; or vivid and uneasy dreams; for example, of animals that bite, of robbers, of unfinished business of the day, bloodshed, death, quarrels, creeping things, and so on. If you walk in your sleep. If you are afraid of the dark and want company.
- Pulsatilla: If you feel wide awake in the evening and your first sleep is restless. You wake feeling languid and unrefreshed. You feel irresistible sleepiness in the afternoon. You sleep with your

hands over your head. If you dislike being covered. If you like to have the window open even though you may be chilly.

- Valeriana: If you experience sleeplessness or disturbed sleep (only able to fall asleep toward morning) with tossing, and anxious and confused dreams.

Homeopathic Remedies for Brain Fog

In relation to brain fog, one of these remedies might fit:

- Kali carb: Poor memory, forgetfulness, mental fatigue and low energy, mind feels dull and sluggish.
- Sepia: Absentmindedness, confusion and thinking difficulties with an indifference to loved ones.
- Phosphoric acid: Inability to collect thoughts or find the right words, rereading the same words and forgetting what is read afterward.
- Anacardium: Marked forgetfulness, dullness of mind and brain fatigue.
- Lycopodium: Confusion, difficulty concentrating on the conversation, difficulty finding the right words, dyslexia, gradual memory loss.

Again, working with a trained homeopath is the best route to find the perfect remedy, as well as the correct dosing structure, that fits your whole symptom picture. However, you can find a wide variety of homeopathic remedies at your local health food store.

Energy Medicine

What is energy medicine? According to Norm Shealy, MD, founding president of the American Holistic Medical Association, "*Energy medicine is the future of all medicine.*"

But what is it, exactly? Well, according to Donna Eden, author/coauthor of five books on energy medicine, "Energy medicine is the term that describes a growing number of approaches where an understanding of the body as a system of energies is being applied for promoting healing, health and well-being." Donna Eden is a pioneer in the field of energy medicine and her work really resonates with me. Her techniques provide the basis of what we are going to talk about here. What I love about energy medicine is that it is simple, easy and free! Once you learn the techniques for moving energy, you can do it anytime, anywhere and address any symptom that you may be experiencing.

One of the fundamental understandings of energy medicine systems is that, in order for health to manifest, your energies need to be able to flow freely and consistently. When energy is stuck, stagnant or flowing in the wrong direction, discomfort, illness, and disease can occur. So, it is vital to make sure your energies are flowing properly on a daily basis.

What can cause energy to become stuck?

- Lack of movement
- Bottled up emotions
- Trauma
- Physical injury
- Sedentary lifestyle

There are many ways to get your energies flowing smoothly again. Some of my favorites are using Donna Eden's Energy Method.

I'm going to go over a quick daily energy routine that I have been following for a few years now. It is based on Donna Eden's 5-Minute Daily Energy Routine. I have found this extremely helpful for keeping my immune system in shape, maintaining consistent energy throughout the day and relieving stress-related symptoms. You can find out more about Eden Energy Medicine here: https://edenmethod.com. I do a little bit of a variation on Donna's routine, but you can find her official version here: https://www.youtube.com/watch?v=Di5Ua44iuXc. I encourage you to practice these along with me as I describe them below.

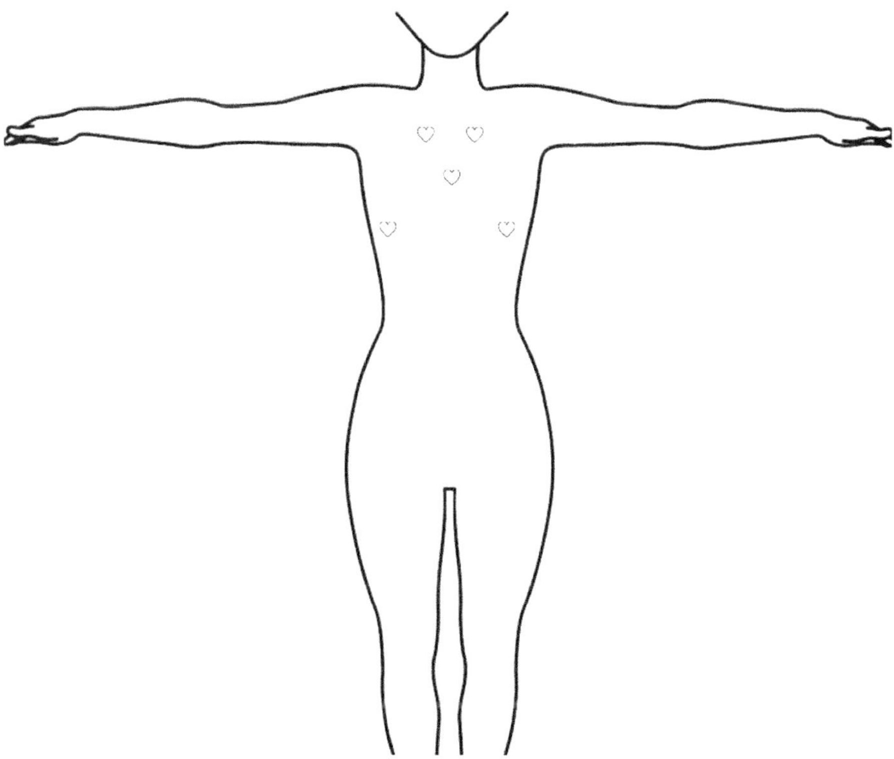

Daily Routine

- Three thumps – K-27, thymus, spleen points
    - Use several fingers or knuckles to tap the spots shown in the picture. Tap vigorously on each set of spots. Focus on breathing in through your nose and out through your mouth during all the tapping.
    - To locate K-27 points, place your fingers on your collarbone and move them inward toward the U-shaped notch at the top of your breastbone. Move your fingers to the bottom of the U and then move down and out about an inch to find the spots. Tap or massage for ten to fifteen seconds.
    - Place the fingers of either or both hands in the center of your sternum at the thymus gland. Tap there for fifteen to twenty seconds with your fingers or your knuckles.
    - Tap the neurolymphatic spleen points, beneath the breasts and down one rib, for fifteen seconds.

Donna says *this energy exercise boosts and restores energy, increases strength and vitality, and strengthens the immune system.*

- Zip up
    - Place your hands at the bottom end of the central meridian – at your pubic bone.
    - Take a deep breath in as you move your hands, slowly and deliberately, straight up the center of your body to your lower lip.
    - Continue upward, bringing your hands past your lips and exuberantly raising them into the sky. Circle your arms

back to your pelvis.

- Repeat three times.
- Zip up this meridian as often as you like.

According to Donna, this b*oosts confidence, clears your thoughts, and protects you from negative energies that may be around you.*

- Hook up
    - Place the middle finger of one hand on the "third eye" (between the eyebrows above the bridge of the nose.
    - Place the middle finger of the other hand in the navel.
    - Gently press each finger into the skin and pull it upward. Hold for twelve to thirty seconds.
    - You can hold it longer if you like.
    - Often you will experience a deep sigh and/or yawn. This shows your energies have hooked up.

According to Donna, *this one gets strange flows moving, strengthens the auric field, and leaves you feeling whole again. It calms and helps you feel connected.*

- Crown pull
    - Place your thumbs at your temples and your fingertips resting at the middle of your forehead.
    - Slowly, with pressure, pull your fingers apart to the hairline stretching the skin above your eyebrows.
    - Place your fingers at the hairline and repeat the stretch.
    - Repeat this pattern starting at the top, center and back of your head. Continue all the way back and down until you

reach the base of your neck. Use pressure as you pull.

- Move down to your shoulders and push your fingers in and hold. Then pull across your shoulders toward the front. Hold your hands there until it feels right, then release and drop your hands/arms.

This one relieves mental congestion and headaches, clears and refreshes the mind, sharpens memory, and opens the crown chakra to higher inspiration.

- Cross crawl
  - While standing, seated or lying down, lift your right arm and left leg simultaneously.
  - As you let them down, raise your left arm and right leg.
  - Repeat, this time exaggerating the lift of your leg and the swing of your arm across the midline to the opposite side of your body.
  - If you can, twist so that your elbow touches your opposite knee.
  - Continue this exaggerated march for at least a minute, again breathing deeply in.

Donna says *this balances and harmonizes energy, improves coordination, and clears thinking.*

I encourage you to adopt a similar routine to start your day, especially if you are experiencing low vitality and energy or any health issues. It's a great way to start addressing your health on a foundational level … and it's kind of fun, too!

It's important to be mindful of our breath when we are doing these energy practices. According to Donna Eden, the lungs can expel 70 percent of the waste from your body. That is why when we start to work with the lungs, powerful changes can happen throughout our body. Although shifting the energy around chronic conditions may take some time, small shifts can happen fast.

Let's Get Specific

Now, let's move on to some specific energy exercises and techniques that can address individual menopausal symptoms:

We're going to start with a liver-clearing energy exercise. You'll remember that we have mentioned in previous chapters how important it is to keep the liver well nourished and well functioning so it can metabolize our hormones properly.

- Liver clearing
    - With your thumb and index finger, massage the webbed area between thumb and index finger.
    - Then massage your hand palm side up and down each finger, ending by bending fingers backward.
- Adrenal stress relief, insomnia relief, hot flash relief, hormone balancing in general
    - Triple Warmer Smoothie:
        - Place fingers at temples and hold one breath. Then slide behind your ears. Down the side of the neck and hang on shoulders. Push fingers into shoulders, drag them over tops of shoulders down to middle of chest, with one arm

resting on top of the other.

- Hot flashes
    - Cool-down acupoint:
        - Press the middle fingers of each hand into a point two inches directly below the navel. Breathe deeply.
- Depression and mental acuity
    - Heart womb connection:
        - Place one hand over the heart chakra and the other over your womb chakra. Notice the two energies connecting – stay for three minutes breathing deeply.

Come back to this section and practice these techniques every day for a week. At that point, you'll be familiar enough with them to be able to incorporate them into your own daily energy rituals.

The Secrets of Energy medicine

ENERGY REMEDIES

Flower Essences

- Walnut
- Cherry Plum
- Olive
- Scleranthus
- Crab Apple

Homeopathic Remedies

Brain Fog
·Kali Carb
·Sepia
·Phosphoric Acid
·Anacardium
·Lycopodium

Hot Flashes
·Lachesis
·Sepia
·Pulsatilla
·Valeriana
·Ferrum metallicum
·Sulfuricum acidum
·Sanguinaria
·Belladonna

Insomnia
·Nux Vomica
·Coffea
·Belladonna
·Chamomilla
·Aconite
·Arsenicum
·Gelsemium
·Phosphorus
·Pulsatilla
·Valeriana

Energy Exercises

- Three Thumps
- Zip Up
- Hook Up
- Crown Pull
- Cross Crawl
- Liver Clearing
- Triple Warmer Smoothie
- Cool-Down Accupoint
- Heart Womb Connection

Which of these forms of Energy Medicine do you feel could help you the most?
Which one do you resonate with and why?

VIBRANT MID-LIFE | Revolution

Chapter 6

Unlock the Magic of Herbs

In this chapter, we are going to learn about what herbal medicine is and why it can be such a critical piece of the puzzle during our midlife journey. Then we are going to cover which specific herbs can address our menopausal symptoms and increase our general level of health.

So, what exactly is herbal medicine? Herbalism is a traditional medicinal or folk medicine practice based on the use of plants and plant extracts. Herbalism is also known as botanical medicine, medical herbalism, herbal medicine, herbology, plant medicine, and phytotherapy. The scope of herbal medicine is sometimes extended to include fungal and bee products, as well as minerals, shells, and certain animal parts. Pharmacognosy is the study of medicines derived from natural sources.

Herbal medicine has been the dominant form of "health care" since the beginning of human culture. Even today, 75 percent of the world's population depends on some form of herbal medicine as their primary source of health care, according to the World Health Organization (WHO).

Herbs are considered nutrient-rich foods and, as such, can be utilized as dietary supplements benefiting anyone regardless of their level of health, as well as complementing and supporting conventional therapy.

Some of the reasons I feel that herbalism has consistently remained so popular worldwide are:

1. Safety – many herbs have been used for centuries and even thousands of years and we have records within several systems of herbal medicine such as Traditional Chinese Medicine and Ayurveda with documented safety data going back almost five thousand years. In contrast, conventional Western medicine has a very poor track record where safety is concerned, with some studies claiming it is the third leading cause of death in the US.
2. Accessibility – most people, no matter where they live, can walk out their backdoor and harvest a dandelion root or grow herbs on their windowsill. Herbal medicine is the people's medicine, accessible to all.
3. Efficacy – again, we have thousands of years of data, in some cases, documenting the effectiveness of plant medicine. In fact, according to research led by Professor Biljana Bauer Petrovsk, the oldest *written* evidence of plant usage for medicinal preparation was found on a Sumerian clay slab from Nagpur, dated approximately five thousand years old.
4. Synergy – our bodies know what to do with plants; they were designed to assimilate their nutrients. Herbal formulations work

> in a subtle manner that is harmonious and synergistic with the body's healing processes. The body's natural defenses are strengthened, allowing the body to heal itself. Herbal remedies don't just alleviate the symptoms of illness but actually work toward fixing the underlying cause of the problem.

There are many different ways to incorporate herbs into daily life. One of the best and most meaningful is to grow them yourself. When you work with plants on a daily basis, you get to know them, their "personalities," and their energies. You begin to get an intuitive feeling for their affinities, what they can offer to you, how they can help you flourish, while, in return, you offer them a healthy place to grow and flourish.

In the goddess culture, Airmid is the Celtic goddess of healing, known as mother of herbal healers, and the world's healing herbs are said to have actually developed from her tears.

Aja is an Orisha (or a human recognized as a goddess). She is another powerful goddess of healing, also known as the spirit of the forest and herbal healers. You are considered to be lucky if you are blessed with her magic, as she holds the secrets of botany and green herbs and tends to pass her skills to the Yoruban people who desired to practice this art.

Before we go further, I want to take a moment to speak to the ancient wisdom that we all hold inside us, the healing wisdom that these goddess traditions allude to. Part of our work is to tap into that intuition and acknowledge the fact that we can be … and are called to be … our own healers at this time in our lives. I'm reminded of a quote from herbalist Rosemary Gladstar:

"I am my own healer.

I have a radiant voice within that guides me.

I can make decisions for myself.

I can rely on others as needed, but at my discretion.

It is my body, my health, my balance, and my responsibility to make right choices for myself. Right choices include working with competent health-care professionals when necessary, allowing friends and family to help as needed, and, above all, being true to my beliefs, with the wisdom and willingness to change as a part of the path of healing."

While herbalism is an art, it is also a science and there are some very fundamental understandings that are important to know when you use herbs as medicine. It is beyond the scope of this book to go deeply into this, but here is a brief primer on using herbal medicine.

Herbal Myths

There are many common myths/misconceptions about herbal medicine. Let's set the record straight.

The first misconception is that all herbs are safe.

- In fact, some herbs are very toxic, and it's important to know which ones are and which ones are not and the appropriate times and ways to use one or the other.

The next myth is that all herbal formulas are safe for everyone.

- Just because an herbal formula exists does not mean it is safe for everyone. Some herbs are safe for adults but not children or babies, and some are not safe for those who are immunocompromised.

The next misconception is that all herbal medicines are free from side effects.

- While the safety data shows that herbal medicine is largely free of side effects, especially when compared to pharmaceutical medicine, some herbs, especially some standardized extracts of herbs, may have side effects you need to be aware of.

Next, herbal products are always pure and natural.

- Unfortunately, the herbal industry is not free from adulteration and marketing gimmicks.

And, finally, my favorite … more is better where herbs are concerned.

- In fact, the opposite is usually true; the least amount that has an effect is usually the best dose to start with.

Now, on to some quick tips regarding how to work with herbal medicine:

Most people just starting out with plant medicine will be purchasing their herbs, so it is crucial to know what to look for.

How to purchase herbs:

- Know and trust your supplier.
- Make sure they smell intensely and fresh.
- Make sure they look vibrant and deep in color.
- Look for organically grown.

After working with plant medicine for a while, you may consider preparing your own herbs.

Why prepare your own herbs?

- You know where they came from.
- You know how they have been handled.
- You know how fresh they are.
- You can infuse your own energy into them.

You may at some point want to start foraging for wild harvesting your own herbs. This is beyond the scope of this book, but I do want to mention the number one rule for gathering your own herbs. This is critical and can be a matter of life and death.

When gathering your own herbs:

- Make sure you have positive ID of the plant to avoid accidentally harvesting a poisonous plant.
- Know which plant part you need.
- Know when that plant part has the most energy.
- Be gentle.
- Avoid any area that could be contaminated.

The next thing you'll need to know is how to store your herbs.

How to store herbs:

- Store in a cool, dark place in an airtight container.
- Avoid light, heat, air, moisture, insects.
- Label with date of harvest and name and check often.
- Make sure they are fully dry before storing them.

And, just briefly, I want to list the various ways you can incorporate herbal medicine into your life, your routine and your rituals.

Applications:

- Teas/tisanes
    - Water infusions
    - Water decoctions
    - Water fomentations
- Poultices
- Tinctures/extracts
    - Alcohol
    - Glycerin
    - Vinegar
- Steam inhalations
- Infused oils
- Salves

Working with Herbs ~ The Basics

An easy to use cheat sheet to get you started using herbal medicine!

Purchasing herbs

- Know and trust your supplier
- Make sure the herbs smell fresh and their aroma is intense
- Make sure they look vibrant and deep in color
- Look for organically grown

Preparing your own

- You know where they came from
- You know how they have been handled
- You know how fresh they are
- You can infuse your own energy into them

Gathering your own

- Make sure you have positive ID
- Know which plant part you need
- Know when that plant part has the most energy
- Be gentle
- Avoid any area that could be contaminated

How to store

- Drying - completely dry before storing: hang in bunches out of direct sun, lay on drying sceens, or use a dehydrator on the lowest setting
- Storing -keep cool, dark and in an air-tight container
- Avoid – light, heat, air, moisture and insects.
- Label - name, harvest date, location

Herbal applications

- Teas/tisanes - Infusions , Decoctions, Fomentations
- Steam Inhalations
- Poultices
- Tinctures/extracts - alcohol, alcohol and water, vinegar or glycerine
- Infused Oils

In the next section, we are going to be talking about how to use herbs as nourishing infusions to provide optimal levels of nutrients to boost your general health and vitality, as well as to address specific menopausal symptoms.

What is a Nourishing Infusion?

Let's break it down:

- Infusion – An infusion is a large amount of herb brewed for a long time. Typically, one ounce by weight (about a cup by volume) of dried herb is placed in a quart jar, which is then filled to the top with boiling water, tightly lidded and allowed to steep for four to ten hours. After straining, a cup or more is consumed, and the remainder chilled to slow spoilage. Drinking two to four cups a day is usual.
- Nourishing – Herbs that make your infusion more nourishing are those that contain lots of minerals and other phytonutrients. The long steeping time extracts many more of the nutrients in the herbs into the liquid that you will be drinking as a tea. Since the minerals and other phytochemicals in nourishing herbs are made more accessible by drying, dried herbs are considered best for infusions.

Beverage Teas VS Nourishing Infusions

What is the difference between a beverage tea and a nourishing infusion? Beverage teas are steeped on average between two and five minutes.

They will have a pleasant flavor and a few benefits for your health, but not much beyond that. Medicinal teas are steeped for around twenty minutes and have many more benefits for your health. The stronger acting herbs are perfect this way. Nourishing infusions are for the food-like herbs that are rich in minerals and phytonutrients and are safe for long-term, daily consumption.

According to herbalist Susan Weed, who made nourishing infusions popular, an infusion is made from a lot of herb (always dry), boiling water and is steeped for several hours. You get all of the above-mentioned plus mineral salts. These mineral salts are bioavailable in wonderful profusion and good balance. Dry herbs are used because drying the plant breaks the cell wall. When the boiling water is poured over them the weakened cell walls open and the mineral salts inside the cells come into the infusion.

Safe Herbs for Nourishing Infusions

Can any herb be prepared as a nourishing infusion? No, only the safest herbs can be used this way. Nourishing herbs are the safest of all herbs. Experiencing any side effects from these herbs is quite rare. In general, nourishing herbs may be taken in any quantity for any period of time. These herbs can be thought of as foods, just as leafy greens, garlic, and mushrooms are. They provide high levels of nutrients including vitamins, minerals, trace minerals, starches, simple and complex sugars, bioflavonoids, carotenes, and essential fatty acids (EFAs). Examples of herbs suitable for nourishing infusions include:

- alfalfa
- borage

- chickweed
- cornsilk
- elder blossoms or berries
- evening primrose
- linden
- mallow
- nettle
- oatstraw
- plantain
- raspberry
- red clover
- seaweeds
- rose hip
- violet

I will go over a few of my favorites for those of us in peri-, mid- and post-menopause in detail.

Oatstraw (Avena sativa)

According to herbalist Susun Weed, a cup of oatstraw infusion contains more than 300 milligrams of calcium plus generous amounts of many other minerals. Its steroidal saponins nourish the pancreas and liver, improving digestion and stabilizing moods.

Oatstraw also contains a high content of iron, manganese, and zinc. It is a tonic for the central nervous system and is highly indicated for those under stress, or those who experience anxiety or depression.

Nettle (Urtica dioica)

A cup of nettle infusion contains 500 milligrams of calcium plus generous amounts of bone-building magnesium, potassium, silicon, boron, and zinc. It is also an excellent source of vitamins A, D, E, and K.

To illustrate the importance of making nourishing infusions from these food-like herbs, a cup of nettle tea, for instance, contains only 5–10 milligrams of calcium, while a cup of nettle infusion contains up to 500 milligrams of calcium.

Throughout Europe, nettle is used as a spring tonic and detoxifying remedy. They support and strengthen the entire body. Nettle builds energy, strengthens the adrenals, is good for breast tenderness due to a build up of hormonal waste and for heavy bleeding.

Linden (Tillia platyphyllos, cordata)

This useful herb contains many flavonoids, gentle nervine relaxant, affinity for the heart – it can calm palpitations and ease anxiety. It is an officially approved medicine in Europe by Commission E for colds and cold-related coughs. According to herbalist David Winston, this herb is a wonderful remedy for mild depression.

Red clover (Trifolium pratense)

This lovely and common herb contains four phytoestrogens and has ten times the amount of phytoestrogens that soy does. Red clover is the world's leading anticancer herb and can improve the memory and is high in antioxidants, especially vitamin E. Red clover is nourishing, vitamin-rich, mineral-rich, containing vitamin B complex, vitamin C, calcium, chromium, magnesium, manganese, niacin, phosphorus, potassium, and protein. It has been successfully used to reduce hot flashes in menopause and may also be beneficial for osteoporosis.

I like to make my infusions at night before I go to bed and then they are ready to drink in the morning. I put my herb in a Mason jar and set the water to boil. Then I pour the boiling water up to the rim of the jar, screw on a tight lid and go to bed.

In the morning, I strain out the herbs and drink the liquid as my nourishing infusion throughout the day. It's wonderful iced, but if I want it hot, I make a beverage tea and add it to my cup of nourishing infusion to warm it up. Drink several cups a day and use it all up because after about thirty-six hours or so it spoils. Then it can be used to water house plants, or poured over hair after washing as a final rinse, which can be left on.

Herbal Love for Your Liver and Adrenals

Specifically, during the menopausal phase of life, there are two main areas it is crucial to support because of the changes in the endocrine/hormonal system, and those are the liver and the adrenals.

Why is the endocrine system so intricately linked to menopausal symptoms? We reviewed the science of how stress affects our hormones, our endocrine system and especially the liver and adrenals in chapter 3 pg 33. You can go back for a quick review.

So, let's look at the liver now. It's critical to support and nourish the liver at this time of a woman's life since the liver is the primary organ used to break down the body's hormones. The liver is often overloaded and sluggish in part because of all the changes the hormonal system is going through during perimenopause, menopause and into post-menopause. This is on top of all the external stressors most women are coping with in midlife. Earlier in the book, we mentioned that women often are going through many changes and shifts in their external lives as well as their internal lives – family changes, relationship changes, careers changes – which all can result in a cortisol spike that has a trickle-down effect on the reproductive hormones, causing fluctuations that the liver has to process. Often, the liver is not able to do its job effectively; it is not able to efficiently metabolize the hormones that the body produces, which can lead to some of the uncomfortable symptoms that we experience in midlife.

Three herbs that are extremely helpful in this area are dandelion, burdock and nettle. Let's take a look at **Dandelion.** We all know this as a pernicious weed in our lawns, but what you may not know is that Dandelion is one of the most used and highly medicinal herbs we have available to us.

- It helps to regulate and balance hormone production through liver strengthening and detoxing
- Both Dandelion leaf and root can help prevent weight gain associated with water retention and the inability to metabolize fat.
- Dandelion is also rich in minerals that help keep bones strong, which is so important in menopausal women.

Burdock! You may know Burdock from the little burrs that get stuck in your pet's fur when walking through the fields or woodlands. But, do you also know that Burdock is one of the best liver herbs there is?

- It has abilities to keep the liver healthy and protected, even from heavy metal toxicity.
- It can reduce liver congestion.
- Because it's a cooling herb, it can calm inflammation and many of the hot conditions that can arise during menopause.

And finally we have nettle. **Stinging Nettle** and I have known each other for a very long time. It is one of my very favorite herbs and I have even found it growing in the southern mountain range in India.

- There are certain compounds produced in the liver that help it to do its job of detoxifying hormones along with everything else. In studies, nettle has been shown to increase the levels of these compounds in the liver.
- It can also protect the liver from toxins and inflammation.
- Nettle is very high in minerals (calcium, potassium, phosphorus, silicon, iron, manganese, sulfur, molybdenum, vanadium), protein and vitamins A, C, D, K.

Next I want to share with you about adaptogens for adrenal support. They work via the HPA axis, which stands for the hypothalamic–pituitary–adrenal pathway of the endocrine system, so they are vitally relevant to our discussion of hormone balance and midlife changes.

Adaptogens are substances that have the ability to help the body adapt to stress. In the past, this category of herbs has been called rejuvenating or restorative herbs, qi tonics or rasayanas. And modern research has proven that these superior herbs, which have such a long tradition of use, are safe and effective.

Andrew Weil, MD, an integrative medicine physician, describes adaptogens as herbs "that can 'tone' the body and bring it back to homeostasis." James Duke, PhD, scientist and ethnobotanist, says, "All plants contain adaptogenic/tonic compounds, because plants have to contend with a good deal of stress themselves." David Winston and Steven Maimes, in their book *Adaptogens, Herbs for Strength, Stamina and Stress Relief,* define adaptogenic herbs as "remarkable natural substances that help the body adapt to stress, support normal metabolic functions and help restore balance." They also outline how the term adaptogen was coined:

> *"In 1947, Dr. Nikolai Lazarev defined adaptogen as an agent that allows the body to counter adverse physical, chemical, or biological stressors by raising nonspecific resistance toward such stress, thus allowing the organism to 'adapt' to the stressful circumstances."*

In 1968, Israel I. Brekhman, PhD, and Dr. I. V. Dardymov formally gave adaptogens a functional definition, as follows:

- An adaptogen is nontoxic to the recipient.
- An adaptogen produces a nonspecific response in the body – an increase in the power of resistance against multiple stressors including physical, chemical, or biological agents.
- An adaptogen has a normalizing influence on physiology,

irrespective of the direction of change from physiological norms by the stressor.

Here is a list of just five of the ways adaptogens can support vibrant health:

1. Help your body adapt to stress via the HPA axis (hypothalamic–pituitary–adrenal).
2. As nontoxic plants they can be used as long-term tonic remedies.
3. Enable the body's cells to access more energy.
4. Mediate inflammatory responses in the body.
5. Regulate endocrine and neuroendocrine balance within the body.

Since stress, inflammation, and endocrine disruption are some of the most foundational and widespread contributors to disease, especially during the menopausal journey, adaptogens might be the perfect addition to your daily health protocol.

"The stress response system – or HPA Axis – is an elegant system. When it gets triggered by a threat it can help you avoid danger, and in an emergency, it's truly lifesaving. But our fight/flight/freeze/fawn response was not meant to stay activated 24/7. When it is, we're in a semi-chronic or chronic state of cortisol and adrenaline overload which can cause an astonishing number of symptoms that women come to see us for, from sleep to digestive to hormonal to mental health to immune-related problems. We need to rest, repair, restore."

– Dr. Aviva Romm

Here are a few examples of herbs that are good adaptogens for menopause:

Ashwagandha is a powerful adaptogenic herb used in Ayurvedic practice.

- It helps to promote mental calm, reduce anxiety, depression, and insomnia.
- In one study, Ashwagandha was shown to increase serum DHEA levels by 13.2 percent. DHEA is the "mother" hormone because it is the precursor of other hormones like estrogen and testosterone.
- So, this is another way Ashwagandha can help balance the hormones during menopause, in addition to helping reduce stress.

Our next adaptogen is **Milky Oats.** This refers to the oat grain when it is still in the fresh, green, milky stage before it matures completely. This herb is a nervous system tonic.

- Milky Oats is specific for any sort of nervous system disorder such as depression, anxiety, shock, tremors, or pain. This also includes nervous exhaustion and mood swings.
- They are high in calcium and magnesium, and phytosterols, which are plant hormones.
- Milky Oats have also been used as an aphrodisiac. Have you ever heard the term sowing your wild oats? This is where it came from.

Next, we have **Tulsi**, or Holy Basil as it is sometimes called.

- As an adaptogen, Tulsi has the ability to regulate cortisol levels and keep your hormone levels balanced naturally.

- Holy Basil calms the adrenals, reduces inflammation, and it increases the sex drive.
- In addition, herbalist David Winston shared that he finds Tulsi helpful as a cerebral stimulant to aid people with poor memory or cloudy thinking, or the "brain fog" that can be experienced by those of us in menopause.

Our next adaptogen is **Maca Root.** The Quechua Indians of Peru consider Maca a food that promotes mental acuity, physical vitality, endurance, and stamina. Aviav Romm, MD, refers to Maca as "the mother of hormone nourishers."

- Maca can help improve low libido.
- It can help resolve or reduce anxiety and depression.
- It is rich in a variety of nutrients, such as essential amino acids, iodine, iron, and magnesium, as well as sterols that may possess a wide range of activities that support adrenal and hormone function.

And, finally, we have **Shatavari.** This is an Ayurvedic herb that is known as the "queen of herbs" and women's adaptogens.

- It is used for irritability and many hormonal imbalances affecting the mood.
- It may be used for vaginal dryness, low libido, and sleep problems in perimenopause.
- Shatavari has mild estrogenic and cholesterol-lowering effects.

There are many herbal adaptogens, but these are ones that are commonly used in menopause and can get you headed in the right direction.

Sleep Better with Herbal Remedies

Earlier in this book, in the foods for sleep section in Chapter 4: Nourish Your Symptoms Away, we spoke about why poor sleep is such a common issue during the menopausal journey.

Many women experience insomnia at various times of their lives. As we enter perimenopause, those episodes of insomnia can worsen for some of us. And, since sleep is when our body rejuvenates, heals and repairs, it is critical to make sure we do everything we can to sleep well on a regular basis.

There are many factors that can result in sleep issues for women in midlife and it is generally necessary to take an individualized approach. However, there are many herbs that can address insomnia stemming from multiple causes:

Lavender (Lavendula ssp.) – Our first sleep herb is lavender. Lavender has long been used to promote relaxation and help prepare our bodies and minds for sleep. While it is commonly used in essential oil form, the plant form can be used to promote sleep as an herbal tea. Lavender is best combined with other herbs in our list, as the taste can be a bit strong for most people.

Chamomile (Matricaria recutita) – A cup of Chamomile tea before bed was a common ritual in days past to relax and send us off into deep, restful sleep. It can be especially helpful if insomnia is a result of anxiety or muscle tension.

Oatstraw (Avena sativa) – We've spoken about Oatstraw before, in the nourishing infusions training. And, while it is not a sedative herb, I have included it here because it is so nourishing to the nervous system. With long-term use , drinking Oatstraw tea provides valuable nutrients that nurture, calm and relax the nervous system and reduce insomnia due to nervous system imbalance.

Skullcap (Scutellaria lateriflora) – This herb has been traditionally used for centuries as a sleep aid. It is gently relaxing and calming. It induces normal sleep without being strongly sedating. It is excellent for insomnia that results from nervousness, anxiety, restlessness or muscular pain and tension.

Passionflower (Passiflora incarnata) – This lovely herb is particularly effective for insomnia with circular thinking or mental chatter. Another benefit is that it not only helps you fall asleep but stay asleep, as well.

Valerian (Valeriana officinalis) – The sedative properties of Valerian have been recognized for over two thousand years! It is beneficial for anxiety, restlessness and pain-induced insomnia. Many herbalists find that upwards of 10 percent of their clients have an opposite reaction to Valerian, so it is wise to test it out to see if it works for you.

Hops (Humulus lupulus) – Hops is best known for its use as the bitter agent in beer making, but hops also has a long history of medicinal use as a sedative, especially when sleeplessness is due to restlessness and anxiety.

California Poppy (Eschscholzia californica) – The California Poppy was used for pain and as a mild sedative by the Pacific coastal American Indian people. It is a gentle, calming and relaxing herb.

While there are many other herbs that can be beneficial for improving insomnia, this is a great place to start.

Slip off to Sleep Herbal Tea

Here is a tried and true recipe for reducing insomnia during the menopausal phase of life:

2 parts Passionflower

1 part Skullcap

1 part Valerian

Steep for 15 minutes and drink 1 cup while winding down in the evening, ½ a cup in the hour before bed and ½ a cup more, if needed, at bedtime. (Be sure to use the bathroom right before bedtime to avoid needing to go in the middle of the night.)

Herbs for Managing Your Moods

Earlier in this book, in the foods for moods section in Chapter 3: Body, Mind, and Spirit: The Key to Radiant Wellness, we spoke about why mood swings, anxiety and depression are such a common issue during the menopausal journey. And we learned that studies show that more than 50 percent of women experience mood swings during the menopausal years. These can include:

- Aggressiveness
- Anxiety

- Depression
- Excessive joy
- Feelings of helplessness,
- Worthlessness, and/or hopelessness
- Irritability
- Sadness

Here are a few medicinal herbs that can help us to balance out our mood swings and reduce our other emotional symptoms:

Oatstraw (Avena sativa) – We've spoken about oat straw not only in the last section on herbs for sleep, but also in our nourishing infusions section ... and we're going to talk about it here too! The oat plant in general is very healing and nurturing to the nervous system, so it can be helpful in improving your moods whether you are eating oatmeal, drinking oat straw tea or taking a milky oats tincture. In fact, milky oats (read more about this part of the oat plant in the herbs for adaptogens section on page 206) are actually considered a nervous system trophorestorative. This means they can actually help rebuild the nervous system.

Nettle (Urtica dioica) – Stinging Nettle is particularly nutrient dense and provides many of the vitamins and minerals our nervous system needs to balance our emotions. It has a particular affinity for the kidneys and adrenals and can be amazingly helpful if your mood imbalance stems from stress and adrenal fatigue.

St. John's Wort (Hypericum perfoliatum) – St. John's Wort is well known as an effective natural antidepressant and recent studies have backed that up, showing comparable effectiveness to several pharmaceutical antidepressant drugs. It is also especially useful for depression caused by seasonal affective disorder when combined with lemon balm.

Motherwort (Leonurus cardiaca) – Is very calming, can help ease nervousness, irritability, anxiety and stress. It is calming, supporting and relaxing to the nervous system. It is also good for heart palpitations, by the way.

Kava kava (Piper methysticum) – The benefits of Kava are an interesting blend of muscle relaxation and mental stimulation and clarity. It relaxes tension while promoting the flow of thoughts. It can help with depression and anxiety.

Dong Quai (Angelica sinensis) – Dong Quai has been used for thousands of years in Traditional Chinese Medicine. One of the ways it can support women in menopause is by helping to stabilize blood sugar, it balances out mood swings and promotes calmness.

Mood Balancing Tincture

Here is a tincture formula for balancing out mood swings, depression and anxiety during the menopausal years.

1 part St. John's Wort
1 part Motherwort
¼ part Dong Quai
Take 1 dropperful 2x/day

Ready made tinctures can be easily found at most health food stores or herb shops. And, while most of the herbs we're discussing are safe for the vast majority of people, it's wisest to work with a trained herbalist, if you are new to herbal medicine.

Herbal Relief for Hot Flashes

Earlier in this book, in the foods for flashes section in Chapter 3: Body, Mind, and Spirit: The Key to Radiant Wellness, we spoke about what a common experience hot flashes are for women in peri-, mid- and post-menopause. It is estimated that up to 80 percent of women will experience hot flashes during the menopausal years and up to 30 percent of them will experience hot flashes and or night sweats for a prolonged period of time. For some, that stretches between seven and eleven years!

Here are a few medicinal herbs that can help us to reduce the frequency, duration and intensity of hot flashes and night sweats:

Red Raspberry leaf (Rubus idaeus) – While most commonly used in pregnancy, when menopausal women use Raspberry leaf, it helps promote healthy uterine tone and minimizes hot flashes. It can also help reduce a heavy flow and is rich in calcium, which supports healthy bones.

Red Clover (Trifolium pratense) – It contains four phytoestrogens and has ten times the amount that soy does. It also contains plenty of nutrients, including vitamins B and C, magnesium and potassium, which can be depleted by hot flashes.

Black Cohosh (Cimicifuga racemosa) – One of the best-studied traditional herbs for menopause, Black Cohosh is used to help alleviate some symptoms of menopause, and is considered an effective hot flash remedy. Black Cohosh seems to work by supporting and maintaining hormonal levels, which may lessen the severity of hot flashes. In studies, it has been proven to be as effective as estrogen replacement therapy.

Motherwort (Leonurus cardiaca) – Can reduce the severity of hot flashes and also night sweats, especially if you take a dose upon awakening with a night sweat. It regulates and tonifies the functioning of the thyroid, blood vessels, liver, heart and uterus.

Fenugreek (Trigonella foenum-graecum) – Rich in protein, essential fatty acids and phytosterols (plant hormones), Fenugreek can greatly reduce the frequency of hot flashes, as well as restore blood sugar balance and increase your libido.

Dong Quai (Angelica sinensis) – Dong Quai has been used for thousands of years in Traditional Chinese Medicine. Dong Quai can very quickly and effectively relieve hot flashes and vaginal dryness. However, if you are a very warm person most of the time, it may make your flashes worse.

Dandelion (Taraxicum officionalis) – Is a superb strengthener for the liver, the control center for hot flashes. Because Dandelion helps the liver to metabolize surplus hormones, it can ease our symptoms, including hot flashes and night sweats.

Ginseng (Panax ginseng) – According to Aviva Romm, MD, Chinese Ginseng taken daily not only reduces hot flashes, but can boost your libido and lower high cholesterol! Take in the early part of the day as ginseng can be stimulating and interfere with sleep.

Cool Down Herbal Tincture

Here is a tincture to help reduce the intensity and frequency of hot flashes during the menopausal years.

1 part Red Clover

1 part Motherwort

1 part Black Cohosh

1 part Dandelion

Take 1 dropperful 3x/day

We covered a number of herbs in this chapter. Please don't feel overwhelmed by all of this information. Go back through the sections and choose just one or two herbs that resonate for you to start experimenting with.

Unlock the Magic of Herbs

HERBAL REMEDIES

Herbs for Mood
- Oatstraw
- Nettles
- St John's Wort
- Motherwort
- Kava Kava
- Dong Quai

Herbs for Sleep
- Lavender
- Chamomile
- Oatstraw
- Skullcap
- Passionflower
- Valerian
- Hops
- California Poppy

Herbs for Flashes
- Red Raspberry lf
- Red Clover
- Black Cohosh
- Motherwort
- Fenugreek
- Dong Quai
- Dandelion
- Ginseng

Nourishing Infusions
- Oatstraw
- Nettles
- Linden
- Red Clover

Adrenal Herbs
- Ashwaganda
- Milky Oats
- Tulsi
- Maca
- Shatavari

Liver Herbs
- Dandelion
- Burdock
- Stinging Nettle

Which of the herbs from this chapter will you incorporate into your own daily ritual to create optimal nutrient uptake and vibrant health?

VIBRANT MID-LIFE Revolution

Chapter 7

Rooting Rituals for Resplendent Daily Living

So what do we do with all this information? In order to utilize it in our lives effectively and make a real difference, we need to integrate it. We need tools and structures that we can use consistently, on a daily basis that will help all our newfound skills, techniques and knowledge take root and flourish in vibrant health.

Movement as a Technique for Transformation

Movement is a powerful way to integrate new habits and learnings into your life, not only to make sure they take root, but to ensure that those roots grow strong and deep. There are many ways to accomplish this:

- Dance
- Natural movement

- Yoga
- Stretching

Release and Integrate Energy

Moving our bodies helps us to release stuck energy. That is one of the reasons we feel so good after dancing for a few minutes or taking a brisk walk. In fact, it is commonly known that an animal's body will shake or tremble after a traumatic incident to help release the energy of the trauma, and therefore, the stress it may cause. And likewise, when we move our bodies intentionally, it helps us to release any blockages of energy that have built up and that allows us to take in new energy. When we are enhancing our personal or spiritual growth, as in the definition of meditation I mentioned in chapter 3, movement can help us move out the old energy and clear the space for the new. Have you ever experienced this? Have you witnessed an animal do this, or have you done it yourself?

Embody the Learning and Healing

There is a hot term right now that explains the next reason I find movement so effective as a form of meditation and integration … and that is embodiment. What is embodiment? One of the definitions is this: *To make part of a system or whole; incorporate.* When we use movement as a meditation, it enables us to incorporate, or make part of our system, the energy of the meditation, or the healing we are receiving or the new concepts we are learning. Movement helps us to embody what we learn, to incorporate and integrate it fully into our entire being.

And it is key to find the type of movement that resonates with you. As a dancer who has studied and practiced various forms of dance, I have found belly dance to be one of the most incredible, sacred embodiment practices there is. What many people don't know is that belly dance is an ancient practice of women's empowerment that was created for a woman's body … to help her navigate the shifts and changes she must make throughout the rhythms and cycles of her life, from first menarche to pregnancy to postpartum to menopause and beyond. It tones and strengthens the pelvic floor, bringing consistent blood flow and keeping her juicy and flexible. It is traditionally performed in community, by women for women and the dance itself tells the story of womanhood. It is body positive and can be learned, practiced and performed by any woman regardless of size, shape or age. I find it to be the perfect embodiment and integration practice for me and many of my clients.

Find YOUR perfect embodiment practice and experience how it helps you integrate your new health and self-care rituals into YOUR life!

Jacqui's Journey Part II

I want to take a moment to tell you a bit more about my client Jacqui. When Jacqui came to me, she had already been living with multiple sclerosis for twenty years and had survived a near-fatal car accident as a young woman, resulting in brain trauma. As a health-care practitioner herself, she had already made many changes in the way she ate, was familiar with herbal remedies and homeopathy. She was fearful of the changes she was experiencing in her body going into perimenopause, particularly brain fog and intense mood swings. One of the things we focused on was creating rituals out of the new tools, remedies and techniques we were creating for her. For example, we co-created a morning ritual that included lighting a beautiful candle, drinking a cup of nourishing infusion (or sometimes miso soup) and taking a few minutes to journal. Jacqui also found that belly dance was integral to elevating her mood, her self-esteem and clarity. She said:

"Midlife seemed like a fairly unknown and frightening dark time … I felt like I was looking at the JIGSAW PUZZLE of my life and there was one big piece missing. What suddenly slotted that 'missing jigsaw piece' into place was the joy of belly dancing classes … I now can feel a whole new sense of purpose just being me. Who and how I am."

– Jacqui

Many ancient cultures used movement as a sacred practice. In Cambodian mythology, the nymph Mera was a "celestial dancer" who married Kambu and founded the nation of the Khmer. To celebrate Mera, ancient Khmer courts staged dances in her honor. Her dance is still popular there today.

Developing New Healthy Habits Through Ritual

We all know and understand that when we make changes in order to improve our lives, they need to become habits, or they just won't stick. We can implement a new way of eating or moving or meditating, but if we don't continue to practice them, we won't see the lasting changes we want. There are a plethora of books written about how to create habits that stick, but very few of them speak to what I find to be one of the best methods to make lasting change in your life … and that is the use of rituals. A very potent and powerful way to integrate new tools and techniques into your life is by creating rituals as a way to habituate yourself to your new healthy routines.

Self-Care Rituals To Embrace The Beauty Within

So, what do I mean by this? In order to be truly healthy, we need to put ourselves and our own needs first. And, in order to do that, we need to know, deep within our hearts, that we are deserving, that we are worthy and that we are loved. For many of us, this is difficult to really, truly feel and embody. We are so busy taking care of others' needs and we don't often feel like we really deserve to put ourselves first.

Fill Your Cup

I think we've all heard the cliche that we need to fill our cup if we want to have anything to give to others. You can't pour from an empty cup, right? Well, I want to take that a step further and say that you can't really give to others in a healthy way, unless your cup is not only full, but overflowing. If your cup is just full (or half full) when you pour out of your cup to nourish the other people in your life, you're once again left with an empty cup. What I want every woman to realize is that her cup needs to be overflowing *all the time.* If your cup is always overflowing, then it's that overflow that can be nurturing all those around you, and yet, you still have a full cup to nurture yourself.

Does this make sense?

Support Your Healing

One way we can ensure our cup is always overflowing is to create self-care rituals. Why rituals? Because they not only help establish the habit, but they are rich and deeply pleasurable. But what stops many of us from having daily or weekly self-care and beauty practices is that we often don't think these kinds of rituals are really going to affect our health in a major way. How is taking care of my skin, or using natural beauty products, going to reduce my symptoms or health conditions? Right? What I would like to suggest is that this is actually the best way to elevate your health and your joy in life. And we have studies to support this.

We know that most of what you put on your body is absorbed into your skin and some of it actually ends up in your bloodstream and your organs.

For example, research shows chemical sunscreen and triclosan in 74.6 percent of individuals tested and phthalates in more than 75 percent. A 2008 study found 16 hormone-altering cosmetics chemicals in teen girls tested and an astounding 287 chemicals in the umbilical cord blood of ten newborn babies. This makes the personal care products you use topically of utmost importance in creating better health. And you have direct control over that.

A recent study in *Diabetologia*, a peer-reviewed medical journal, sheds light on the relationship between these common and ubiquitous exposures of forever chemicals and women's metabolic health:

"Women in midlife exposed to combinations of perfluoroalkyl and polyfluoroalkyl substances (PFASs), dubbed 'forever and everywhere chemicals,' are at increased risk of developing diabetes, similar to the magnitude of risk associated with overweight, and even greater than the risk associated with smoking." Further: "1.5 million Americans are newly diagnosed with diabetes each year in the USA, approximately 370,000 new cases of diabetes annually in the US are attributable to PFA exposure."

We also know that how we feel about how we look – whether we feel beautiful or not – affects not only our confidence but our health outcomes. Negative body image has been scientifically linked to depression, anxiety, increased pain sensitivity, and affects quality of life in all areas.

And, we know that when we ritualize things – when we make them into a habit that is meaningful for us – we are much more likely to keep doing them, and then those rituals are much more likely to make a bigger impact on our lives over time. In fact, a 2019 study in the *American Journal of Lifestyle Medicine* concluded that health-care providers can greatly improve patients' chronic disease management, by helping them build a routine around the lifestyle changes that they need to make.

Let's do a small beauty ritual right now together, so we can get an experience of just how simple and nurturing it can be.

Avocado Mask

Why an avocado mask? Avocados are fairly easy for most people to find, they are easy to use as a mask, and they have quite a few benefits for the skin:

- First, the unique monounsaturated fatty acid content allows the avocado to reach deep into your pores. Therefore, they provide a deep cleanse for your skin.
- Secondly, they not only hydrate the skin but enrich it with antioxidants and minerals. That helps to reduce skin sagging and reduces oxidative stress.
- Avocados contain vitamins A, E, and K omega-3 fatty acids.
- This all means they can clean, moisturize, rejuvenate, and heal your skin!

Slice off a small piece of your avocado and scoop the flesh into a small bowl. With a spoon, mash the avocado flesh into a smooth consistency. With your fingers, smooth your avocado paste all over your face, being careful to avoid the eye area. Give yourself a nice, light facial massage while you do this. Leave it on your skin for about ten minutes, then wash off with cool water and moisturize! How simple is that?!

You can create a more complex recipe by adding honey, olive oil or an egg white, or you can just use avocado!

How does your skin feel after your avocado mask?

Soft? Silky? Glowing?

You can make a weekly self-care ritual out of that avocado mask.

Here is another self-care ritual that I use every morning:

The Oil Cleansing Method

A brief overview of my favorite facial cleansing technique:

- Wet a washcloth with hot water, wring it out and lay it over your face for a minute or two.
- Freshen your cloth with hot water, repeat and then gently massage your face with the cloth to loosen any dirt and makeup.
- Warm a teaspoon or two of facial oil (jojoba is a great one to begin with) in the palms of your hands and thoroughly massage your face, taking care to be extra gentle with the delicate skin around the eyes.
- Wet your washcloth again with hot water, wring out and lay over your face.
- Gently wipe away any dirt and makeup that the oil has loosened from your skin.
- Leave the remaining oils on your face to soak in and moisturize.

And here is an example of how you can take several of the exercises and practices we've covered previously and create a nurturing stress-reducing self-care ritual out of them:

Ten-Minute Nurture Pause

We all need a little reminder to practice good self-care routines. But, so often I hear from women, and have experienced myself, that even though we have good intentions, we can't seem to find the time to put them into practice on a regular basis. One reason is that we tend to think that taking care of our own needs will take up a large portion of our time. We are stretched in so many ways today that even the thought of adding one more thing to our schedule, even if it is something that is enjoyable or relaxing, seems overwhelming and unmanageable.

It doesn't have to be that way, though. Self-care doesn't have to take a lot of time. Sure, it's great to spend a day at the spa or carve out a few hours in the evening for a relaxing mineral soak in the tub. But there are many more rituals and techniques that we can add to our self-care toolbox that can be done with a minimal amount of time and effort.

I propose creating a ten-minute nurture pause that you can use at least once a day, and perhaps even more often. It can give you a chance to physically, mentally and emotionally shift into a calmer, more relaxed and focused space, which can have long-lasting positive effects on your mood and health, especially if you create the intention to use this practice long term. Here are a few ideas of what you might include in your ritual:

A cup of herbal tea:

Setting a cup of tea to steep at the beginning of your ten minutes can give you time to go through the rest of your ritual and come back to enjoy your tea at the end. Depending on your needs for the day, your choice of tea could be something relaxing such as chamomile or passionflower, or something stimulating such as rosemary or holy basil.

Deep breathing:

There are many different breathing techniques that can be explored to assist you in your self-care routine. From breathing light into any area of your body where you are feeling pain or discomfort, to focusing on your breath as you practice belly breathing, to specific techniques such as progressive relaxation breathing, bellows breath, or Sudarshan Kriya, practicing breathing exercises can not only relieve stress and restore calm and balance, but also improve the functioning of the immune and nervous systems.

Aromatherapy:

A really easy way to use aromatherapy simply and effectively is to keep a diffuser in your house or on your desk at work. When you are pausing your day to practice your self-care routine, it takes just a moment to turn it on and fill your space with a lovely, healthy aroma. Again, depending on your needs for that day, you might choose a relaxing, stress-relieving oil such as lavender, or an energizing oil like peppermint or lemon.

Being present:

> *"The secret of health for both mind and body is not to mourn for the past, nor to worry about the future, but to live the present moment wisely and earnestly."*
>
> – Buddha

Practicing presence exercises is an amazingly effective way to help us shift from stress or overwhelm to a state of peace and contentment. Being present, or practicing mindfulness, can help clear the mind, bring a sense of gratitude, build inner peace, unleash creativity, and improve physical, mental and emotional health. A simple mindfulness exercise is called Using Your Senses. To practice this exercise, take a moment to consciously pay attention to the world around you through all your senses. What do you see? What do you hear? What can you smell, taste or feel in this moment?

Walk outside:

Just stepping outside can change our mood, clear our mind and enable us to look at things with a fresh perspective. Additionally, even a short, brisk walk on a regular basis can improve circulation, lower blood pressure, aid in weight loss, and enhance immune function.

Which of these ideas resonate with you?

Which ones will you include in your ten-minute nurture pause?

What other ideas do you have for creating your own ritual of self-care?

Nurturing Meno-Morphosis with Support and Accountability

In our modern world, and especially now that our world is more virtual than ever, one of the things we are missing is connection. It is so important to have someone who is your cheerleader, your support system, with whom you can share similar struggles, celebrations, successes and challenges. When our societies were more tribal or village-like we had a built-in support system. Now we need to create that for ourselves. This is crucial. We all need support to be our best and to face our challenges head-on.

As women, we crave community and connection. It is one of the facets and strengths of our feminine energy. We are meant to be *interdependent,* but unfortunately, today's culture celebrates an unbalanced sense of masculine energy and rewards independence and going it alone. Especially as we travel the menopausal journey and undertake the metamorphosis of this phase of our lives, being proactive in securing the support we need and nurturing a strong community of compassionate women to surround us with love and caring is nonnegotiable.

Motivation and inspiration are two of the most critical components of creating change in our lives and making new, healthy habits stick. Accountability is one way we can use motivation and inspiration. When we are not only accountable to ourselves, but others as well, we create a feedback loop of motivation that naturally encourages us to remember why we are working to make changes in our lives and creates inspiration by building support directly into that structure. Being accountable to ourselves and each other can make all the difference in being inspired to create new, healthy rituals that shift us from challenge and struggle into ease and joy!

So now it's time to put all of these tips, tools and techniques together and activate your Vibrant Midlife Goddess Plan! My deepest wish is that this plan will accelerate your Meno-Morphosis so you can step into your wise woman years with confidence, vibrant health and radiant energy and create a passionate, fulfilling and impactful second spring!

Rooting Rituals for Resplendent Daily Living

INTEGRATION

.In this chapter we talked about talked about many ways to integrate everything we've covered so far into your life:

- Movement/Embodiment
- Developing habits through ritual
- Support
- Accountability

How will you use each of these to integrate? How often? In what way?
Make a note of them below.

VIBRANT MID-LIFE Revolution

Chapter 8

Activate Your Vibrant Midlife Goddess Plan

You've reached the last chapter in the book! This is a big milestone and I invite you to take a moment to celebrate all you have learned, implemented and accomplished …

Take a minute to bring to mind at least one thing from each chapter that was the most interesting or pertinent for you and why.

In the next section we are going to be using some of these takeaways to anchor in all we've learned and build your unique path forward to create your Vibrant Midlife Goddess Plan!

You've come a long way and you deserve to honor yourself in a way that is meaningful to you. So, take a moment right now to reflect on all of the new healthy rituals you have created for yourself throughout this program and all the shifts and transformations you've experienced as a result.

Take a deep breath and still your mind. Allow gratitude to fill your body with each inhalation you take and stay in this moment of gratitude for as long as it feels good to you. When you are ready, open your eyes, find a sheet of paper or journal (or use the worksheet below) and write down as many accomplishments, results and transformations you've experienced since you began reading this book as you can think of.

This can include new healthy eating habits, movement routines, meditation rituals, mindset reframes, aha moments, takeaways and any positive results you are experiencing in your life on the physical, mental, emotional and spiritual levels.

Your Vibrant Mid-Life Goddess Plan

Gratitude Journaling

Take a deep breath and still your mind. Allow gratitude to fill your body with each inhalation you take and stay in this moment of gratitude for as long as it feels good to you.

When you are ready, open your eyes and write down as many accomplishments, results and transformations you've experienced in our time together, that you can think of. This can include new healthy eating habits, movement routines, meditation rituals, mindset reframes, aha's, takeaways and any positive results you are experiencing in your life on the physical, mental, emotional and spiritual levels.

VIBRANT MID-LIFE | Revolution

Then, I invite you to use the next activity, Writing your New Story, to bring to mind some of your former health and lifestyle choices that did not serve you. Write down that old story … for example, perhaps you were locked into an unhealthy pattern of eating or negative thinking that resulted in negative consequences for your health. Write that old story down and how it affected your life.

Then take that old story, and over a heat-safe bowl or cooking pot, ideally in an outdoor setting, ask to release yourself from this old destructive story and light the paper on fire and drop it into the bowl. As it burns, ask to release this old story, your old negative habits or mindsets, and purify and heal them so you can move forward in renewed health and vibrancy.

Your Vibrant Mid-Life Goddess Plan

WRITE YOUR STORY

Bring to mind some of your former health and lifestyle choices that did not serve you. **Write down that old story**...for example, perhaps you were locked into an unhealthy pattern of eating or negative thinking that resulted in negative consequences for your health. Write that old story down and how it affected your life.

Then, over a heat safe bowl or cooking pot, ideally in an outdoor setting, ask to release yourself from this old destructive story and light the paper on fire and drop it into the bowl. As it burns, ask to release this old story, your old negative habits or mindsets, purify and heal them so you can move forward in renewed health and vibrancy.

VIBRANT MID-LIFE | Revolution

Then, on the next part of the worksheet, write your new story. Your story of wellness, radiance and your vibrant midlife. Write the details of the new rituals that now serve you in healthy ways to elevate you, to support you and encourage you to use your unique gifts to step into your power in this next chapter of your life. Include the items from your accomplishments list you created in the previous worksheet.

Use this simple ceremony to seal in your intentions for moving forward on your Vibrant Midlife Goddess Plan. Post your new story somewhere where you can see and read it daily.

Perhaps make that part of one of your new healing rituals?

Write your new story... Your story of wellness, radiance and your vibrant mid-life. Write the details of the new rituals that now serve you in healthy ways to elevate you, to support you and encourage you to use your unique gifts to step into your power in this next chapter of your life.

Include the items from your accomplishments list you created in the previous worksheet. Use this simple ceremony to seal in your intentions for moving forward on your Vibrant Mid-Life Goddess Plan. Post your new story somewhere where you can see and read it daily. Perhaps make this part of one of your new healing rituals?

VIBRANT MID-LIFE | Revolution

To make these releasing and intention rituals even more powerful, you can do the releasing part (the old story) on the full moon and the intention setting part (new story) on the new moon. Then be observant of how it was for you.

How did it feel to release?

What dropped in for you as you set your new intentions?

In this section we will be pulling together everything we've done in all the previous chapters to create your unique Vibrant Midlife Goddess Plan so that you can move forward with clarity, radiance and confidence!

The first step is to go back to Chapter 2, Menopause Is Your Spiritual Initiation, and find your worksheets entitled What's Your Why, Follow Your Bliss, and your Food Mood Journal. Refresh your memory by going over your answers on these worksheets and then go through your Food Mood Journal to make any correlations between what you are eating and doing and what symptoms you have been experiencing, if you haven't done that already throughout the program. Pay special attention to how your symptoms may have changed after you started incorporating suggestions from the chapters along the way.

Your next step is to download the Vibrant Midlife Goddess Plan because you will be using it to create your path forward in the next steps. (https://www.herbsofgracehealingarts.com/goddess-plan)

Vibrant Mid-Life Goddess Plan

Start Here

Mind/Body/Spirit

- [ ] Mindfulness
- [ ] Meditation
- [ ] Breathwork
- [ ] Presence
- [ ] Gratitude

Deep Nourishment

- [ ] Food as Medicine
- [ ] Foods for Healthy Weight
- [ ] Foods for Flashes
- [ ] Foods for Sleep
- [ ] Foods for Moods
- [ ] Foods for Brain

Continue

Everything is Energy

- [ ] Flower Essences
- [ ] Homeopathy
- [ ] Energy Medicine

Magic of Herbs

- [ ] Nourishing Infusions
- [ ] Herbs for Sleep
- [ ] Herbs for Moods
- [ ] Herbs for Flashes
- [ ] Adaptogens
- [ ] Liver Herbs

End Here

YOUR VIBRANT MID-LIFE GODDESS PLAN

Now, go back to Chapter 3, Body, Mind, and Spirit: The Key to Radiant Wellness and find your worksheets entitled Daily Mindfulness Practices through Thought, Breathwork, Presence and Gratitude. Review the answers you wrote at the time and which ones you have actually put into practice. Mark the ones that you have resonated with the most and have been the most helpful on your Vibrant Midlife Goddess Plan in the integrating mind/body/spirit section.

The next step is to go back to Chapter 4, Nourish Your Symptoms Away and find your worksheets. Review the answers you wrote at the time and which ones you have actually put into practice. Mark the ones that you have resonated with the most and have been the most helpful on your Vibrant Midlife Goddess Plan in the deep nourishment section.

Now go back to Chapter 5, The Secrets of Energy Medicine and find your worksheets. Do the same thing with these worksheets – Review your answers and which ones you have actually put into practice. Mark the ones that you have resonated with the most and have been the most helpful on your Vibrant Midlife Goddess Plan in the everything is energy section.

The next step is to go back to Chapter 6, Unlock the Magic of Herbs and find your worksheets. Again, review your answers and which ones you have actually put into practice. Mark the ones that you have resonated with the most and have been the most helpful on your Vibrant Midlife Goddess Plan in the magic of herbs section.

Now you have all the pieces of your plan all together in one easy-to-use document. This is your unique Vibrant Midlife Goddess Plan! You only need to refer to this plan any time you need encouragement or a reminder of all the things that are working together to elevate your vitality and well-being.

Your last step is to retake the Meno-Morphosis Midlife Assessment (https://forms.gle/1Q6hgA2SHddcX8ps6) and compare it to the one you took at the beginning of the book to see just how far you have come since then and how much improvement you have experienced in all the areas of your health.

Congratulations! You have completed your Vibrant Midlife Goddess Plan! What an accomplishment. I'm so proud of all the work you've put into your health and the incredible transformations you've experienced. Here's to your vibrant midlife!

Appendices:

I. Recipes

II. Resources

III. Food Charts

IV. Materia Medica

V. Rituals

Recipes

Vanessa's Morning Energy Green Drink

- 12 oz green tea steeped 15–30 minutes
- ½ fresh squeezed lemon juice
- ½ fresh squeezed lime juice
- 1 handful of fresh parsley
- 2 tsp liquid chlorophyll
- glassful of ice cubes
- optional: other herbal teas in addition to green tea, such as maca root, red clover, medicinal mushroom powder (I like lion's mane and reishi) or milky oat tops and a handful of dried parsley

Add all ingredients to blender and blend until it is all liquified and you no longer see flecks of parsley. I based this recipe on a similar one I learned from Dr. D. Lindsey Berkson, so I would like to give her proper recognition.

Traditional Sauerkraut

Traditionally fermented, homemade sauerkraut is not only a culinary delight but a big boost for your health!

Most store-bought sauerkraut is not fermented the traditional way and does not contain the billions of probiotics that the real stuff does. So skip the store-bought and do it yourself! Making your own sauerkraut is simple and easy. Here is a quick tutorial for how to make your own sauerkraut at home:

For my favorite recipe, you will need 1 head of cabbage, a couple cloves of garlic and a tablespoon of sea salt.

- Finely chop or shred the entire head of cabbage.
- As you shred, pack it into a glass canning jar, sprinkling a little sea salt and mixing it in as you go.
- If you'd like, you can also mince some fresh garlic and add that to the mix. I usually use about 2 or 3 large cloves per head of cabbage.
- Using a wooden spoon or pounder, pack the cabbage, salt and garlic down for about 10 minutes or until the juice starts to rise above the level of the vegetables. Make sure none of the vegetables are sticking up out of the juices.
- Leave the lid slightly open to release the pressure from the build up of gasses as your sauerkraut ferments, or open every day to let it escape.

You can start taste testing after a few days. I like to ferment my cabbage for about 4–6 weeks, but some people prefer a milder ferment. Eat a bit with every meal – or at the very least once a day.

* Extra tip – Use organic cabbage and garlic to benefit the health of the planet as well as your own!

* Bonus tip – You can use almost any vegetable to make sauerkraut. One of my favorites is carrots with ginger!

Cilantro Pistachio Pesto

- 1 cup packed fresh cilantro leaves (substitute any combination of fresh nettle, dandelion greens, etc.)
- ½ cup shelled pistachios
- ½ cup olive oil

- ½ cup parmesan cheese
- 6 cloves garlic, peeled
- zest of one lemon
- sea salt to taste

Place all ingredients in a food processor and blend.

Herbal Feta Dip

- 8 oz cream cheese, softened
- 8 oz yogurt
- 6 oz crumbled feta cheese
- 4 large cloves garlic, peeled and minced
- 1 tsp dried nettle
- ½ tsp basil
- ½ tsp oregano

Place all ingredients in a bowl and mix thoroughly.

Northwest Fiesta Salsa

- 5 medium tomatoes
- ½ large onion
- ½ yellow bell pepper
- 6 cloves garlic
- 1 large bunch cilantro
- 3 dandelion leaves
- 1 tbsp dried nettle leaves
- 10 fresh viola leaves

- 1 small bunch of cleavers
- juice of 1 small lime
- sea salt to taste

Place all ingredients in food processor and blend.

Herbal Snack Balls

- ½ cup nut butter
- ¼ cup maple syrup
- ¼ cup raw honey
- 1 tbsp powdered cinnamon
- 1 tsp powdered ginger
- 1 tsp powdered acerola cherry
- 1 tsp powdered rose hip
- ¼ tsp powdered cloves
- 1/16 tsp powdered cayenne
- ½ cup raw cacao powder

Mix the nut butters and sweeteners. Then mix in the powdered herbs. Then add the cacao powder and mix thoroughly. Roll into balls. Finally, roll balls in cacao powder.

Herbal Dark Chocolate Truffles

- 4 oz of 100% powdered cacao
- 4 oz of bittersweet chocolate chips
- ⅔ cup heavy organic cream
- 2 tsp vanilla extract

- 1 tsp powdered cinnamon
- ½ tsp powdered nutmeg
- ½ tsp powdered nettle leaf
- dash of powdered cayenne
- powdered cacao and powdered rose hips for rolling

Place cacao and chocolate chips into a medium-sized bowl along with the vanilla, powdered cinnamon, nutmeg, nettle and cayenne. Warm the cream slowly until just before it starts to simmer. Pour this immediately into the bowl with chocolate. Let this stand for one minute and then stir with a whisk until the chocolate is melted and it has a smooth consistency. Cool the truffle sauce to a semihard consistency in the fridge or freezer and check it frequently. It needs to be soft enough to form into a ball yet hard enough to roll without falling apart. Once the desired consistency is reached you can start rolling. Scoop the mixture into bite-sized pieces and, using clean hands, roll into a ball. Then roll the balls in the powder.

Baked Amaranth Vegetable Patties

- 1 cup dry amaranth
- 2 cups water
- 1 tbsp coconut oil
- 1 medium onion, minced
- 2 medium carrots, grated
- 2 medium zucchini, grated
- 3 cups fresh swiss chard, finely chopped
- ¼ cup gluten-free flour mix
- ½ tsp baking powder

- 3 tbsp tahini
- 3 handfuls fresh herbs, finely chopped
- juice of ½ lemon
- 1 tsp sea salt
- black pepper

Place the amaranth and the water in a pot. Bring to a boil, cover and simmer for 20 minutes until amaranth is soft and water is absorbed. Remove lid, fluff and set aside to cool. Preheat oven to 400°F. Line a baking sheet with parchment paper and then lightly oil. In a pan, sauté onion in oil. Add carrots and zucchini and sauté until all is soft. Add swiss chard and cook just until wilted. In a large mixing bowl, mix amaranth, cooked veggies and all remaining ingredients. Mix with your hands until it is all uniformly combined. Taste and adjust seasonings to your liking. Shape mixture into about 10 patties and place on baking sheet. Bake 20–30 minutes until golden and crunchy on the top. Serve as is or topped with a dab or your favorite sauce.

Sun-Dried Tomato, Mushroom, and Swiss Chard Frittata

- 1 tbsp coconut oil
- 1 leek thinly sliced
- 3 large garlic cloves, minced
- 3 cups (8 oz) sliced cremini mushrooms
- ½ cup fresh chives, finely chopped
- ½ cup fresh herbs, finely chopped
- ⅓ cup oil-packed sun-dried tomatoes, finely chopped
- 1 cup swiss chard

- 4 eggs
- 1 cup raw milk or cream
- ½ cup raw cheddar cheese
- ¾–1 tsp fine grain sea salt
- black pepper, to taste

Preheat oven to 400°F. In a cast iron skillet, add oil and sauté the leek and garlic over medium heat for a few minutes. Stir in the mushrooms, season with salt, and cook on medium-high heat until most of the water cooks off the mushrooms, about 10–12 minutes. Stir in the herbs, sun-dried tomatoes, swiss chard, salt, pepper, and red pepper flakes until combined. Cook until the swiss chard is wilted. In a bowl, combine eggs and milk/cream until well mixed. Add the veggies to the egg mixture and stir. Add more oil to skillet and then pour mixture back in. Sprinkle cheese on top. Cook until bottom is just golden brown, then transfer to over for 5–10 minutes until golden brown on top.

Herbal Butternut Squash Soup

- 2 large butternut squash
- melted butter for brushing
- 1 large onion
- 1 large head of garlic
- 1 tbsp coconut oil
- 1 tsp ginger
- 1 tsp turmeric
- 3 cups of overnight nettle/oat straw/alfalfa infusion
- 4 tbsp honey

- ½ cup nut milk
- sea salt and pepper to taste
- dash nutmeg

Preheat the oven to 400°F. Cut the squash lengthwise. Brush the flesh of the squash with butter and season with 1 tablespoon salt and 1 teaspoon pepper. On a sheet pan lay the squash flesh side up. Roast for about 30 to 35 minutes or until the flesh is nice and soft. In the meantime, sauté onion, and garlic in the coconut oil in a large pot. Scoop the flesh from the skin of the squash into the pot and add the infusion, honey, turmeric and ginger. Bring to a simmer and puree using a stick blender. Stir in the heavy cream and return to a low simmer. Season with salt, pepper, and nutmeg.

Black Bean Chili

- 2 tbsp coconut oil
- 1 onion
- 6 cloves garlic
- 1 large carrot
- 1 red bell pepper
- 2 tbsp cumin
- 1 tbsp each oregano, sage, thyme
- dash of cayenne
- sea salt and pepper to taste
- red pepper flakes to taste
- 1 can diced tomatoes
- 3 cans black beans

Sauté diced onion, garlic, carrot and pepper in the coconut oil until tender.

Add herbs and continue to salute for a few more minutes.

Add tomatoes and beans. Cook over medium heat for 20 minutes.

Fire Cider

Fire cider (also called master tonic sometimes) is one of my favorite winter remedies for several reasons. First, it's very effective; made with ingredients such as garlic, ginger and cayenne, it is seriously antimicrobial, anti-inflammatory and detoxifying.

Second, the apple cider vinegar that is the medium for this concoction is not only a great preservative, so it will keep for a long time, but it has a plethora of health benefits itself, such as killing bacteria and soothing inflammation. Last, and perhaps best, is that it is so easy to make!

Here's a step-by-step tutorial showing you just how simple it is to make your own cold and flu prevention remedy, so you can be prepared for the winter season:

- Mince garlic, onion, ginger, cayenne, turmeric and any other ingredients you would like to add, such as horseradish, rosemary or oregano.
- Add all ingredients to a clean glass jar. I've also added a bit of black pepper since it helps the other ingredients to be more bioavailable.
- Cover the ingredients with apple cider vinegar by about an inch. The ingredients may float to the top at first.

- Place lid tightly on jar and store in a dark, cool place. Shake daily for a few weeks.

That's it! Easy-peasy! Once the mixture has macerated for a few weeks, you can start using the liquid. You can do that either by straining out the chunks, or, if you're like me, just leave them in and pour the liquid off the top when you need it. Take a spoonful, diluted in water, every day for prevention. Or, if you are already sick, take it every few hours.

Kichari

- 1 cup mung beans
- 1 cup basmati rice
- 9 cups water
- 4 cups chopped vegetables
- (carrot, celery, green beans, broccoli, etc.) 1/2 c coconut oil
- 2 onions, chopped
- 1/3 cup minced ginger root
- 8-10 cloves garlic, minced
- 1 heaping t. turmeric 1/2 t. black pepper
- 1 t. curry powder
- 1 t. crushed red chili 1/2 t. cumin powder
- 2 bay leaves
- Seeds of 5 cardamom pods Salt to taste
- Chopped cilantro leaves

Wash beans and rice. Bring water to boil, add rice and beans, and let boil over medium high. Prepare vegetables. Add vegetables to cooking rice and beans. Heat oil in a large frying pan. Add onion, ginger and garlic.

Sauté over medium high until translucent. Add turmeric, black pepper, curry and red chili. When nicely well done, combine onion mixture with cooking beans and rice. Stir often to prevent scorching. Add remaining ingredients. Continue cooking until totally and completely well done, over medium high, stirring often. The consistency should be rich, thick, and soupy. Serve topped with cilantro and/or yogurt over the top.

Resources

RECOMMENDED READING LIST

Herbal Medicine - General

A Modern Herbal Volumes 1 & 2 – Maude Grieve
Foundations of Health – Christopher Hobbs
Nature's Children – Juliette de Bairacli Levy
The Illustrated Herbal Handbook for Everyone - Juliette de Bairacli Levy
Herbal Body Book – Jeanne Rose
Herbs and Things - Jeanne Rose
The Complete Medicinal Herbal - Penelope Ody
Herbally Yours – Penny C Royal
Herbal Medicine – Rudolph Weiss
Wise Woman Herbal: Healing Wise – Susun Weed
The Earthwise Herbal: A Complete Guide to New World Medicinal Plants – Matthew Wood
The Earthwise Herbal: A Complete Guide to Old World Medicinal Plants – Matthew Wood
The Book of Herbal Wisdom: Using Plants as Medicines – Matthew Wood
The Green Pharmacy – James Duke
Practical Herbs – Henriette Kress
Rosemary Gladstar's Medicinal Herbs: A Beginner's Guide – Rosemary Gladstar
The Herbalist's Way: The Art and Practice of Healing with Plant Medicines – Michael & Nancy Phillips
The Herbal Medicine-Maker's Handbook: A Home Manual – James Green
Herbal Medicine From the Heart of the Earth – Sharol Tilgner

Herb Safety

Botanical Safety Handbook - American Herbal Products Association
Herb Contraindications and Drug Interactions -Francis J Brinker
Drug-Herb-Vitamin Interactions Bible -Steven Bratman, Richard Harkness

Recommended Reading List

Herbs for Family/Children/Women/Men

Herbal Healing for Women – Rosemary Gladstar
The Family Herbal - Rosemary Gladstar
The Male Herbal – Jim Green
Wise Woman Herbal: Herbal for the Childbearing Year – Susun Weed
Wise Woman Herbal: Menopausal Years – Susun Weed
Breast Cancer? Breast Health! The Wise Woman Way - Susun Weed
Down There: Sexual and Reproductive Health The Wise Woman Way - Susun Weed
Botanical Medicine for Women's Health – Aviva Jill Romm
Naturally Healthy Babies and Children – Aviva Jill Romm
Women's Herbs, Women's Health – Christopher Hobbs and Kathy Keville
A Kid's Herb Book – Lesley Tierra
Hygieia: A Woman's Herbal – Jeannine Parvati

Ethnobotony

Ethnobotony of Western Washington – Erna Gunther
Indian Herbology of North America – Hutchens
Medicinal Plants of Native America – Daniel Moerman
Native American Ethnobotany - Daniel Moerman

NorthWest Plants

Medicinal Plants of the Pacific West – Michael Moore
Plants of the Pacific NorthWest Coast - Pojar & Mackinnon
Wild Rose and Western Red Cedar – Elise Krohn
Edible and Medicinal Plants of the West – Gregory Tilford

Recommended Reading List

Plant Identification

A Field Guide to Pacific States Wildflowers – Theodore Niehaus
Field Guide to Edible Wild Plants – Bradford Angier
A field Guide to Western Medicinal Plants and Herbs – Christopher Hobbs, Steven Foster

Herbal Cultivation

Growing 101 Herbs That Heal – Tammi Hartung
A Grower's Guide to Herbs - Geoffrey Burnie and John Fenton-Smith
The Medicinal Herb Grower – Richo Cech

Advanced/Specialized Herbalism

Medical Herbalism: The Science and Practice of Herbal Medicine – David Hoffman
The Earthwise Herbal Repertory: The Definitive Practitioner's Guide – Matthew Wood
Adaptogens: Herbs for Strength, Stamina and Stress Relief – David Winston and Steven Maimes
Healing Lyme Disease Coinfections – Stephen Harrod Buhner
Dental Herbalism: Natural Therapies for the Mouth – Leslie Alexander and Linda Straub-Bruce
Herbal Constituents: Foundations of Phytochemistry - by Lisa Ganora
The Practicing Herbalist: Meeting With Clients ~ Reading the Body - by Margi Flint

Recommended Reading List

Online Herbal Resources

Michael Moore/SW School of Botanical Medicine: http://www.swsbm.com/
Native American Ethnobotany: http://herb.umd.umich.edu/
Herb Mentor: http://www.herbmentor.com/
Home of the electronic version of "A Modern Herbal" by Maud Grieve: http://botanical.com/
Herbalist Jim McDonald's site: http://www.herbcraft.org/seedsstems.html
Herbalist Henriette Kress's site: http://www.henriettesherbal.com/
Herbalist Matthew Wood's site: http://www.matthewwoodherbs.com/
Articles by Herbalist David Hoffman: http://www.herbcraft.org/hoffmann.html
Susun Weed's website: http://www.susunweed.com/
Washington Herbalist Ryan Drum's site: http://www.ryandrum.com/
Herbalist Kiva Rose's site: http://bearmedicineherbals.com/
Herbalist 7Song's site: www.7song.com
Herbalist Paul Bergner's site: www.naimh.com
Herbalist Todd Caldecott's site: www.toddcaldecott.com
James Duke -Medical Botany www.ars-grin.gov/duke/syllabus
Herbalist Sharol Tilgner's site: www.herbaltransitions.com
Herbalist Howie Brounstein's site: www.botanicalstudies.net
Herbalist Rosalee de la Forêt's site: www.methowvalleyherbs.com
Herbalist Christopher Hobbs's site: www.christopherhobbs.com
Organic Medicinal herb seed company: http://www.horizonherbs.com/
Certified Organic herb seller: http://www.mountainroseherbs.com/
Certified Organic herb seller: http://www.pacificbotanicals.com/
Botanical drawings: http://luirig.altervista.org/photos-search/
Breitenbush Herbal Conference: http://www.breitenbushherbalconference.com/
Traditions in Western Herbalism Conference:http://www.traditionsinwesternherbalism.org/
Dandelion Seed Conference: http://www.oly-wa.us/DandelionCollective/PastEvents.php
Portland Plant Gathering: http://www.pdxplantmedicine.org/wp/
CommonWealth Herbs Reading List: http://commonwealthherbs.com/CWH-apprenticeship-readings.html
The Plant List: http://www.theplantlist.org/

Recommended Reading List

Homeopathy

Organon of Medicine: The Classic Work on Homoepathy – Samuel Hahnemann
Discovering Homeopathy – Dana Ullman
The Consumer's Guide to Homeopathy – Dana Ullman
The Complete Homeopathy Handbook - Miranda Castro
Homeopathy for Pregnancy, Birth and Baby's First Year – Miranda Castro
The Homeopathic Treatment of Children – Paul Herscu
Yasgur's Homeopathic Dictionary
Portraits of Homeopathic Medicines – Catherine R. Coulter

Homeopathic Repertories and Materia Medicas

Prisma: The Arcana of Materia Medica Illuminated – Frans Vermeulen
Repertory of the Homeopathic Materia Medica – J.T. Kent
Pocket Manual of Homeopathic Materia Medica and Repertory – William Boericke
A Dictionary of Practical Materia Medica 3 Volumes – John Henry Clarke

Homeoprophylaxis

Homeopathy in Epidemic Diseases – Dorothy Shepherd
A Handbook of Homeopathic Alternatives to Immunisation – Susan Curtis
The Complete Practitioner's Maual of Homeoprophylaxis – Dr Isaac Golden
The Solution: Homeoprophylaxis: The Vaccine Alternative - Kate Birch and Cilla Whatcott

Recommended Reading List

Aromatherapy

The Aromatherapy Practitioner Reference Manual – Sylla Sheppard-Hanger
Essential Oil Safety: A Guide for Health Care Professionals -Robert Tisserand and Rodney Young
The Art of Aromatherapy- Robert Tisserand
The Aromatherapy Book – Jeanne Rose
The Practice of Aromatherapy – Jean Valnet
Medical Aromatherapy – Kurt Schnaubelt
Making Aromatherapy Creams and Lotions – Donna Maria
Hydrosols - Suzanne Catty

Online Aromatherapy Resources

Appalachian Valley Natural Products -BEST Essential Oils- (http://av-at.com/)
Liberty Natural Products (www.libertynatural.com/)
Green Mountain Organics (http://www.greenmountainorganics.com)
Quality essential oils: http://www.mountainroseherbs.com/

Flower Essences

The Bach Flower Remedies – Edward Bach and F. J. Wheeler
Handbook of the Bach Flower Remedies – Philip M. Chancellor
Bach Flower Remedis to the Rescue – Gregory Vlamis
Bach Flower Remedies for Children – Barbara Mazzarella
Flower Essence Repertory – Patricia Kaminski and Richard Katz
Flower Power – Anne McIntyre

RECOMMENDED READING LIST

Nutritional Therapy

Principles and Practices of Naturopathic Clinical Nutrition – Jonathan Prousky
Food as Medicine – Todd Caldecott
Encyclopedia of Nutritional Supplements – Michael T Murray
The Healing Foods Cookbook – Editors of Prevention Magazine
Common Sense Diet and Health – Svevo Brooks
Nourishing Traditions – Sally Fallon
Prescription for Nutritional Healing - Phyllis Balch, and Dr. James Balch

Reflexology

Complete Reflexology for Life –Barbara Kunz
Hand and Foot Reflexology: A Self-Help Guide- Kevin Kunz and Barbara Kunz
The Complete Guide to Reflexology by Ruth Hull
An Introductory Guide to Reflexology by Louise Tucker
Reflexology The Definitive Practitioners Manual by Beryl Crane
The Reflexology Handbook by Laura Norman

Energy Medicine

Energy Medicine – Donna Eden
Energy Medicine for Women – Donna Eden
Vibrational Medicine – Richard Gerber

Recommended Reading List

Misc Online Resources

GreenMedInfo: http://www.greenmedinfo.com/
Healthy People, Healthy Planet: http://www.healthy.net/
National Center for Homeopathy: http://www.homeopathycenter.org/
http://holisticonline.com/
Homeopath Miranda Castro's website: http://www.mirandacastro.com/
Homeopath Dana Ullman's website: https://www.homeopathic.com/
Homeopathy International: http://www.homeoint.org/english/
Homeopath Luc De Shepper's website: http://www.drluc.com/
Washington Homeopathic Products: http://www.homeopathyworks.com/

Food Charts

Prebiotics:

- acacia gum (or gum arabic)
- raw asparagus
- raw chicory root
- raw dandelion greens
- raw garlic
- raw honey
- raw Jerusalem artichoke
- raw jicama
- raw leeks
- raw or cooked onions
- underripe bananas

Probiotics:

- beet kvass
- buttermilk
- dosa
- kefir (water and milk)
- kimchi
- kombucha
- lassi
- miso
- natto
- raw cheeses
- raw milk
- sauerkraut

- sourdough
- soy sauce
- tempeh
- yogurt

Phytoestrogens:

- alfalfa sprouts
- aniseed
- apples
- barley
- beetroot
- brewer's yeast
- broad beans
- broccoli
- brown rice
- bulgur wheat
- cabbage
- carrots
- celery
- cherries
- chickpeas
- citrus
- clover
- corn
- couscous
- cucumbers
- dried apricots

- dried dates
- garlic
- green beans
- green split peas
- green squash
- hummus
- kidney beans
- legumes
- linseed
- mung bean sprouts
- nuts
- oats
- olive oil
- olives
- papaya
- peas
- plums
- poppy seeds
- potatoes
- pumpkin seeds
- red onions
- rhubarb
- rye
- sesame seeds
- soy
- squash
- sunflower seeds
- sweet peppers

- tofu
- tomatoes

Vitamin C:

- acerola cherries
- amla
- berries
- broccoli
- Brussels sprouts
- cantaloupe
- cauliflower
- citrus
- dandelion leaf
- kiwi
- peppers
- pineapple
- rose hip
- spinach
- tomatoes
- violet leaf and flower

Vitamin E:

- asparagus
- avocado
- broccoli
- dark leafy greens
- eggs

- nuts
- plant oils
- salmon
- seeds
- squash
- trout

Vitamin B:

- dark leafy greens
- brown rice
- polenta
- buckwheat
- nuts and seeds
- organ meats
- sweet potatoes
- avocados
- egg yolks
- fish
- whey

Vitamin D:

- butter
- cheese
- cod liver oil
- egg yolk
- fish
- mushrooms

- yogurt

Minerals:

- Potassium:
    - cabbage
    - celery
    - seaweed
- Iodine:
    - leafy greens grown in gardens fertilized with seaweed
    - mushrooms
    - seaweed
    - unrefined sea salt
- Iron:
    - chocolate
    - liver
    - red meat
    - seaweed
- Calcium:
    - beans
    - dark leafy greens
    - legumes
    - raw nuts and seeds
    - tempeh
- Magnesium:
    - almonds
    - brazil nuts
    - brown rice

- cashews
- chocolate
- kidney beans
- pecans, rye
- swiss chard
- soybeans

Bitter foods:

- apple cider vinegar
- artichoke
- arugula
- bitter melon
- broccoli rabe
- Brussels sprouts
- coffee
- cranberries
- dandelion greens
- dark chocolate
- eggplant
- endive
- grapefruit
- kale
- saffron
- sesame seeds

Omega-3 fatty acids:

- chia seeds
- cod liver oil
- fish such as mackerel, salmon, and herring
- flaxseed
- oysters
- walnuts

Healthy fats:

- avocado
- coconut oil
- grass-fed organic butter
- nuts
- olive oil
- wild-caught salmon

Antioxidants (lutein, zeaxanthin and anthocyanins):

- avocado
- blackberries
- blueberries
- collard greens
- kale
- mustard greens
- raspberries
- spinach
- strawberries

Materia Medica for Midlife

Oatstraw/Milky Oats (Avena sativa)

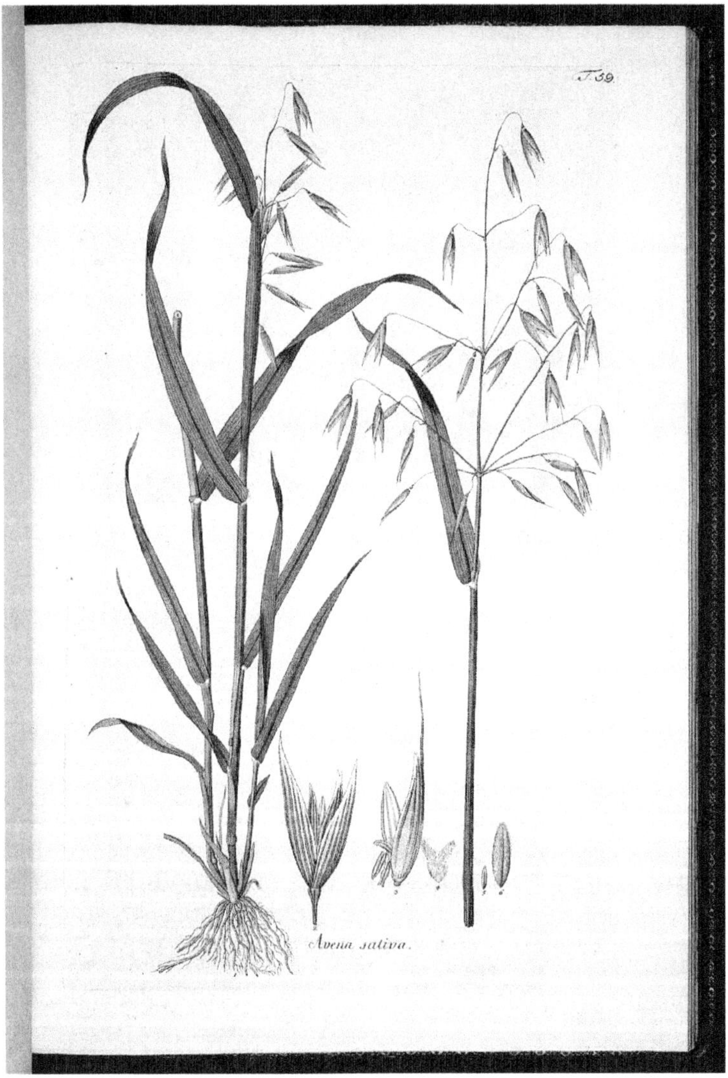

- The oat plant in general is a very healing and nurturing tonic for the nervous system, so it can be helpful in improving your moods whether you are eating oatmeal, drinking oat straw tea or taking a Milky Oats tincture. In fact, Milky Oats (which refers to the top of the oat plant when it is in the milky stage just before the oats mature) are considered a nervous system trophorestorative … that means it can actually help rebuild the nervous system and the myelin sheath that protects the nerves.
- Milky Oats is specific for any sort of nervous system disorder such as depression, anxiety, shock, tremors, or pain. This also includes nervous exhaustion and mood swings.
- Oats are high in calcium and magnesium, and phytosterols (remember we talked about phytoestrogens when we were speaking about using foods as medicine). Phytosterols are plant hormones.
- Milky Oats have also been used as an aphrodisiac … have you ever heard the phrase "sowing your wild oats" … this is where it came from.
- Fresh Milky Oat tops, taken long term, may help regenerate the hippocampus (translating experience into a narrative, verbally and artistically).
- A good mineral tonic and totally nontoxic, steel-cut cooked oats are a good way to use them … or whole grain oats cut in a blender.
- According to herbalist Susun Weed, "A cup of Oatstraw infusion contains more than 300 milligrams of calcium plus generous amounts of many other minerals. Its steroidal saponins nourish the pancreas and liver, improving digestion and stabilizing moods."
    - Oatstraw also contains a high content of iron, manganese, and zinc

- Strengthens and increases flexibility of bones and teeth
- Can help stabilize blood sugar levels
- Relieves depression and mood swings
- Improves circulation
- Nourishes nervous system and helps relieve stress
- Can help improve sleep quality
- Eases urinary and vaginal disturbances

Stinging Nettle (Urtica dioica)

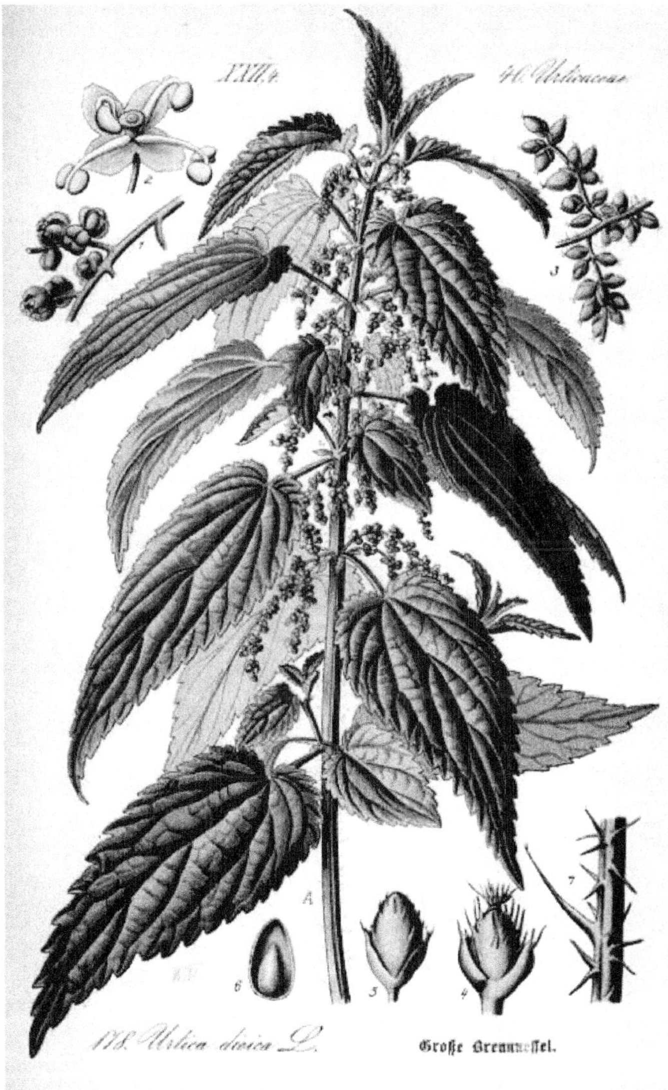

- Throughout Europe, Nettle is used as a spring tonic and detoxifying remedy. It supports and strengthens the entire body. Nettle builds energy, strengthens the adrenals, is good for breast tenderness due to build up of hormonal waste and for heavy bleeding.
- Nettle is very high in minerals such as calcium, magnesium, potassium, silicon, boron, and zinc. It is also an excellent source of vitamins A, D, E, and K.
- To illustrate the importance of making nourishing infusions from food-like herbs such as stinging Nettle, a cup of nettle tea, for instance, contains only 5–10 milligrams of calcium, while a cup of nettle infusion contains up to 500 milligrams of calcium.
- Nettle helps the detoxification process of the liver, while also protecting the liver from inflammation.
- Because of its high mineral and iron content, it is recommended for replenishing the body after blood loss and prolonged illness. For the same reason it is often used as an iron tonic and in anti-anemia formulas.
- Adding a little vinegar or lemon to a stock pot helps to extract minerals from any dark green leaf, such as Nettle.
- Pick when it is young and tender, dry it, keep it dry, and harvest before it flowers. After it flowers, it may irritate the urinary system.
- For addressing hay fever symptoms, start taking nettle daily at least one month before the symptoms begin.
- Nettle is often used as a diuretic for hypertension and other venous insufficiency cases; an anti-inflammatory for arthritis, rheumatism, gout, and so on, both internally and externally; it's good for allergies; it is also hypo- and hyperglycemic.
    - Very good plant source of iron and protein

- Can nourish and rebuild kidneys and adrenals (esp. the seeds), improving energy and stamina
- Eases cystitis and incontinence
- Helps rehydrate vaginal tissues
- Nurtures and strengthens bones, teeth and hair
- Helps heal and support the digestive and immune systems.

Red Clover (Trifolium pratense)

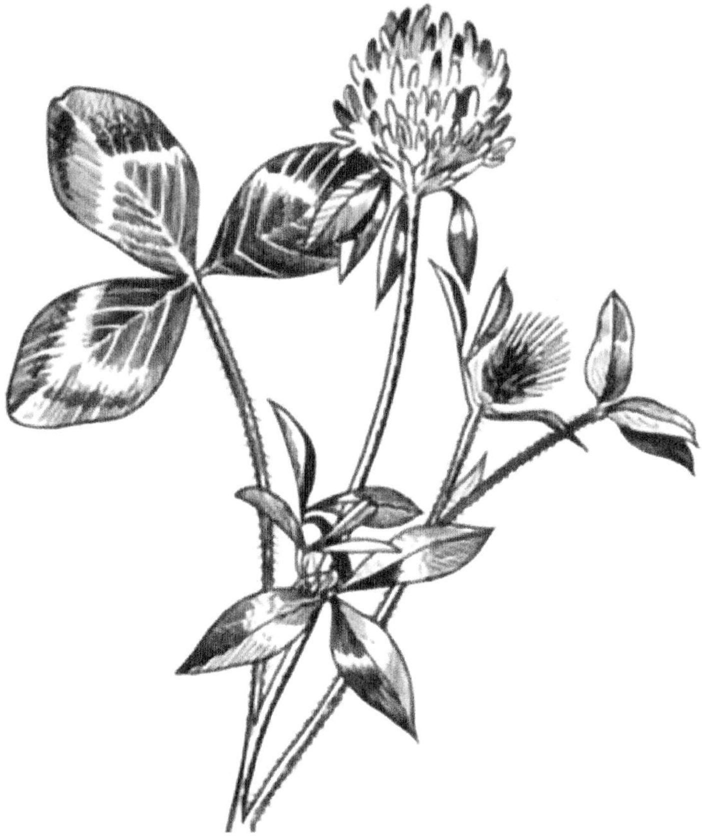

- Red Clover contains four types of phytoestrogens and has ten times the amount that soy does.
- It is one of the world's leading anticancer herbs and has been used to address cancer and other tumors for centuries.
- Red Clover is nourishing, vitamin-rich, mineral-rich, containing vitamin B complex, vitamin C, calcium, chromium, magnesium, manganese, niacin, phosphorus, potassium, and protein. It is also high in antioxidants, especially vitamin E.
- It has been successfully used to reduce hot flashes in menopause and may also be beneficial for osteoporosis.
    - May calm sore joints, anxiety, and fatigue
    - May thin the blood (helpful for stroke prevention, but do not use if flooding)
    - Can help improve the memory

Dandelion (Taraxacum officinale)

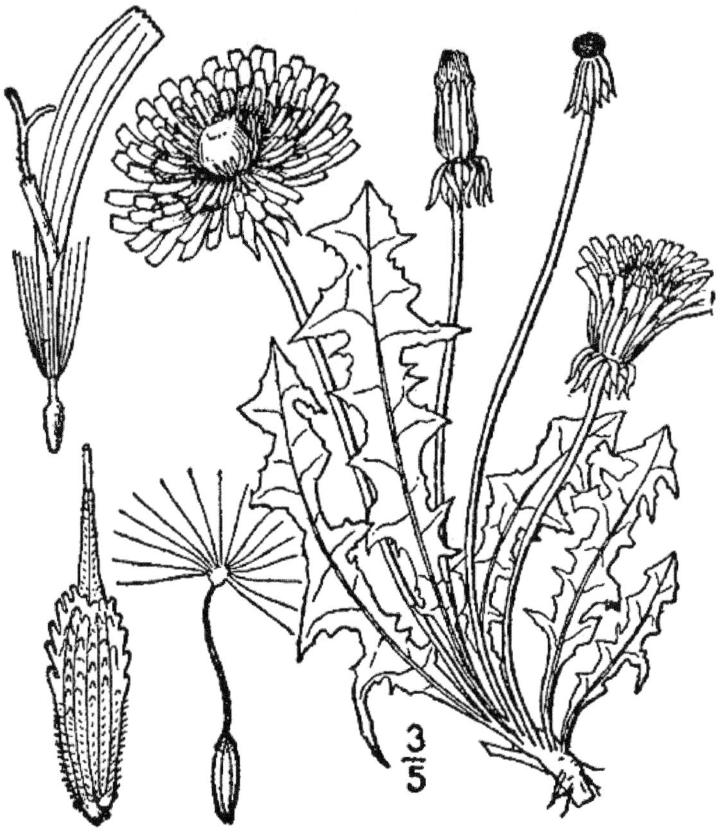

- Dandelion helps to regulate and balance hormone production through liver nourishing and detoxing.
- Both Dandelion leaf and root can help prevent weight gain associated with water retention and the inability to metabolize fat.
- Dandelion is also rich in minerals that help keep bones strong, which is so important in menopausal women.
- A dependable bitter, stimulating digestion, with a particular affinity to the kidneys and liver; it stimulates cell metabolism in those large glands as well as connective tissue; specific for gallbladder disease, rheumatic complaints and degenerative joint diseases. As a liver strengthener and nourisher, it helps relieve food allergies as well as repairs damage from drugs/ infections.
- Dandelion is known to stop the promotion of oncogenes. (When damaged or turned on, an oncogene initiates cancer.) Helps keep breasts healthy, reverses cancerous changes. Helps the liver to make high-quality fats versus low, and is also helpful for diabetics in normalizing blood sugar production.
- Dandelion is a superb strengthener for the liver, the control center for hot flashes. Because Dandelion helps the liver to metabolize surplus hormones, it can ease our symptoms, including hot flashes and night sweats.
    - Can strengthen bones by improving calcium absorption
    - It is high in plant estrogens
    - Rich in vitamins A & C, iron, calcium, potassium and trace minerals
    - Good for hypertension and as a cholagogue (increases the flow of bile)
    - The leaves can be used along with the roots

Burdock (Arctium lappa)

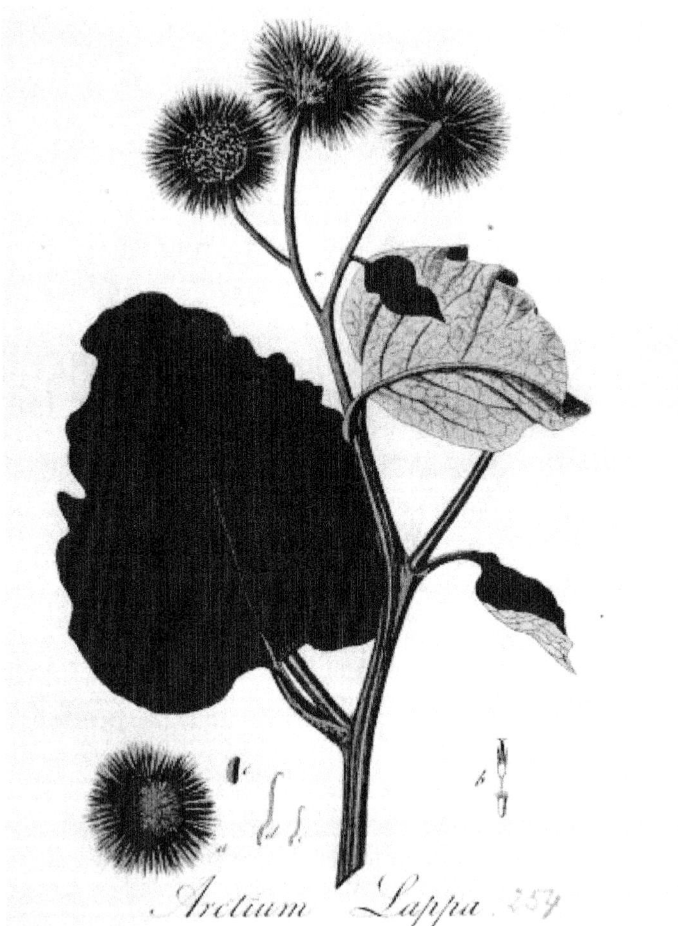

- The root of the Burdock plant has been used as both food and medicine throughout history.
- It has abilities to keep the liver healthy and protected, even from heavy metal toxicity.
- Because it's a cooling herb, it can calm inflammation and many of the hot conditions that can arise during menopause.
- Burdock is regarded as a blood or liver tonic to help detoxify the body. It may be slightly laxative, as well as help lower blood sugar levels.
- It can help reduce liver congestion, and it was used in many old-fashioned cancer remedies.

Ashwagandha (Withania somnifera)

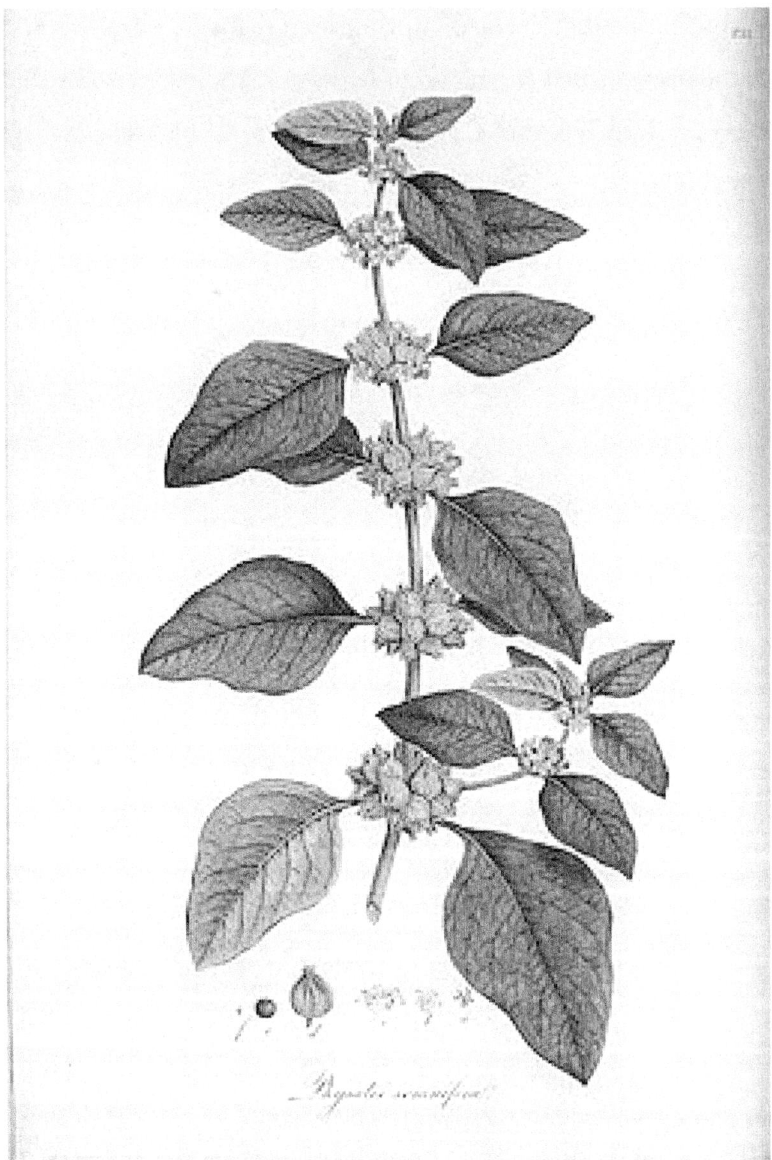

- Ashwagandha is a powerful adaptogenic herb that has been used in Ayurvedic practice for centuries.
- It aids in reducing stress by helping to promote mental calm, reducing anxiety, depression, and insomnia.
- In one study, Ashwagandha was shown to increase serum DHEA levels by 13.2 percent. DHEA is the "mother" hormone because it is the precursor of other hormones like estrogen and testosterone. So, this is another way Ashwagandha can help balance the hormones during menopause, in addition to helping reduce stress.

Holy Basil (Ocimum tenuiflorum)

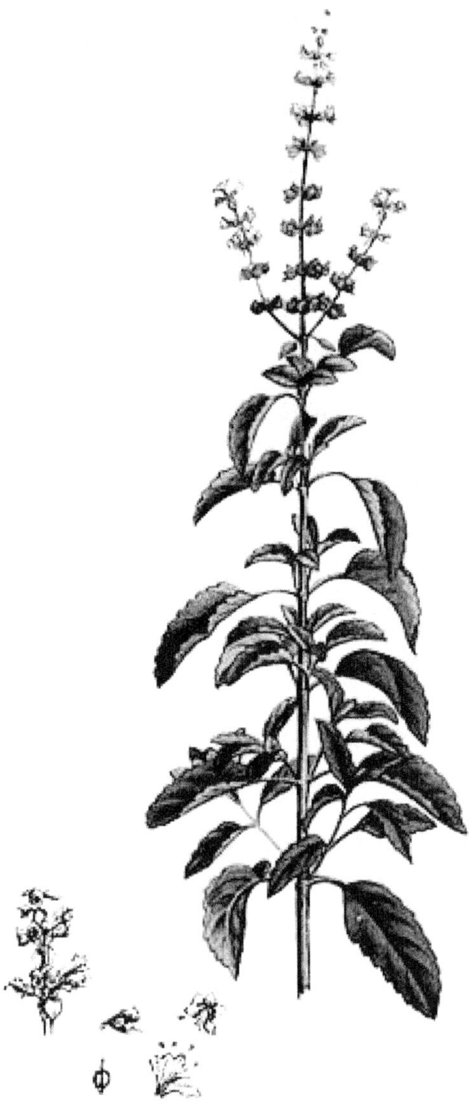

- As an adaptogen, Holy Basil has the ability to regulate cortisol levels and keep your hormones balanced naturally.
- Holy Basil will calm the adrenals, it can reduce inflammation, and it can increase the sex drive.
- In addition, herbalist David Winston shared that he finds Holy Basil helpful as a cerebral stimulant to aid people with poor memory or cloudy thinking, or the "brain fog" that can be experienced by those of us in menopause.

Motherwort (Leonurus cardiaca)

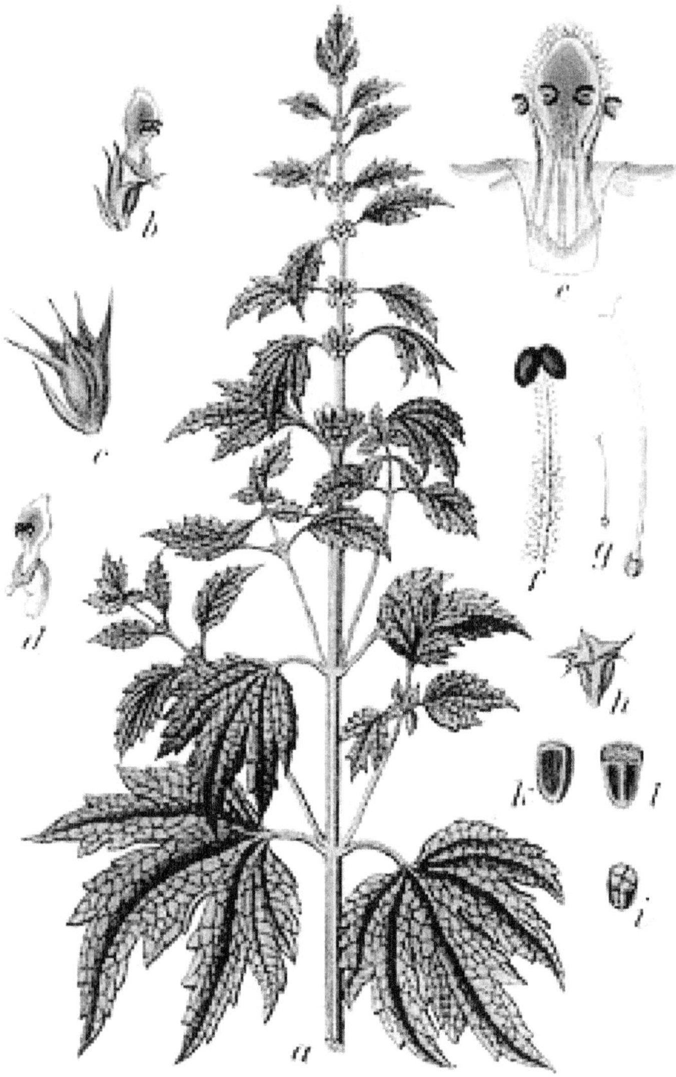

- Motherwort benefits the heart, the circulatory system and women's reproductive health.
- It is an herb for lowering blood pressure, slowing a rapid heartbeat, and calming hormonal mood swings.
- Motherwort may help calm menstrual pain by reducing spasms in the uterus as well as improving blood flow to the pelvis.
- It is especially indicated where anxiety and insomnia are also part of the symptom picture.
- A Chinese legend claims that a sage who drank a cup of Motherwort tea everyday lived to be over three hundred years old.

Sage (Salvia officinalis)

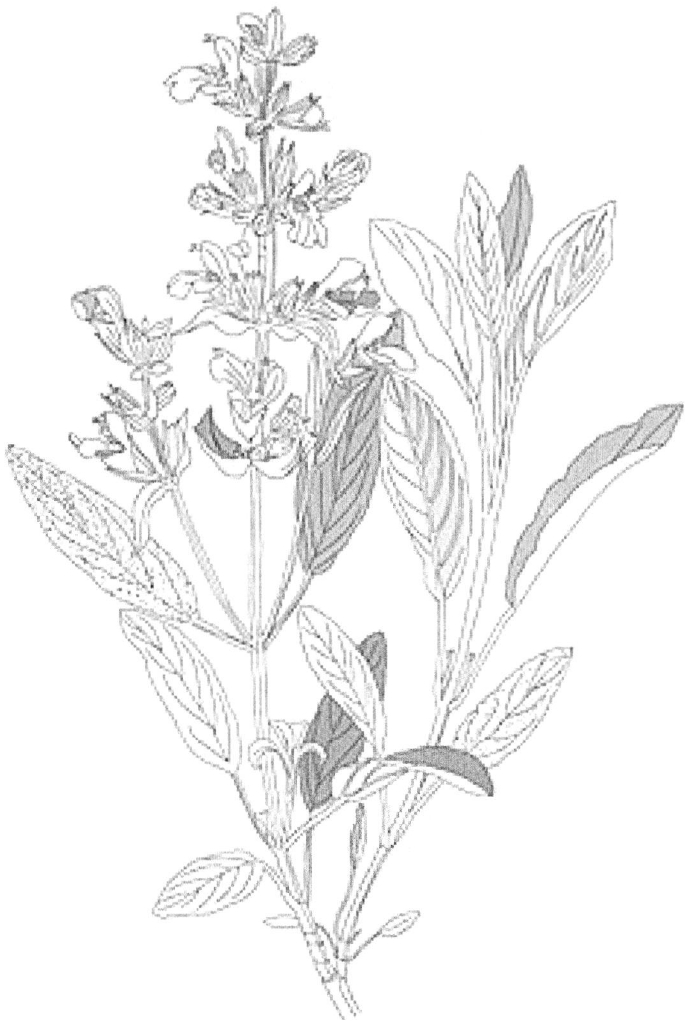

- The antiseptic nature and antioxidant content of sage help slow the aging process, preventing wrinkles and gray hair.
- Sage also has been shown to help prevent cancer and support a calm, focused mind.
- Sage has the property of being a bit drying and this is part of the mechanism by which studies show Sage can help eliminate hot flashes and night sweats.
- It helps regulate hormones, which can ease nerves and decrease depression.
    - Aids digestion, bloating and gas
    - Relieves menstrual cramping and flooding
    - Sage is helpful especially in digesting fats
    - Sage can be helpful for breast conditions and suppresses lactation

Chaste Tree (Vitex agnus castus)

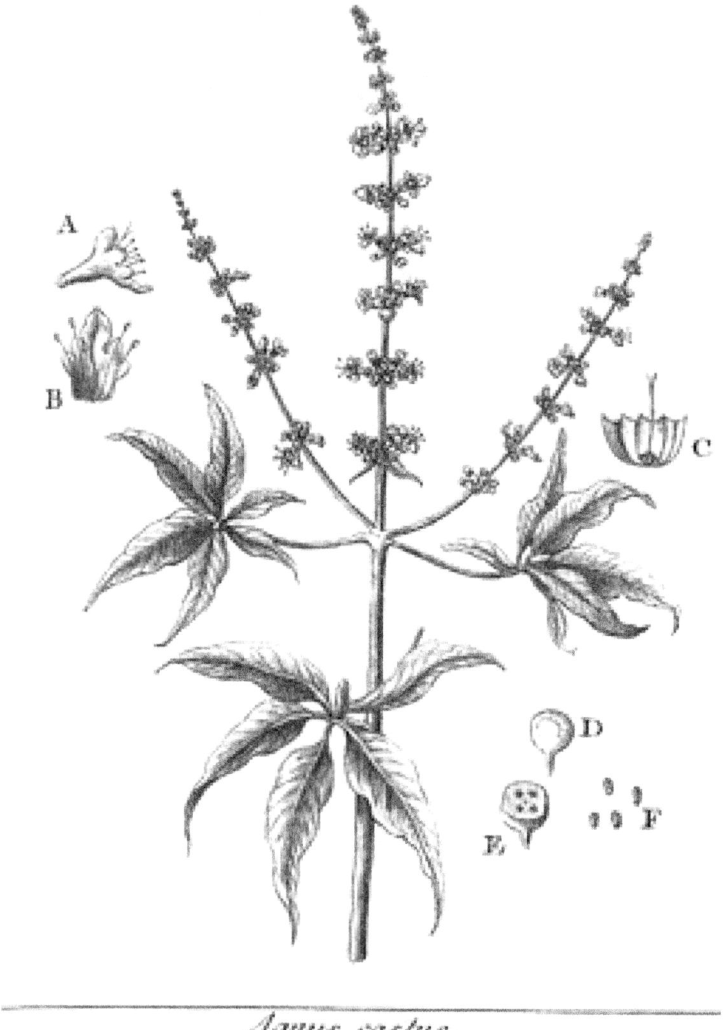

- Vitex stimulates the pituitary gland, which regulates hormone production, so this makes it invaluable for balancing our hormones, especially during perimenopause.
- Studies show that it can enhance the progesterone cycle. At the same time, it restores the estrogen/progesterone balance.
- One of the ways Vitex is helpful during the menopausal phase is that it can redirect nutrition toward the reproductive cycle.
- One study found a 93 percent decrease in PMS symptoms when taking Vitex.
- A study of one hundred women found that Vitex was able to cut monthly migraines in half in 42 percent of the patients, and a total of 57 women had fewer headache days.
    - Helpful for fibrocystic breasts, irregular menses, infertility, fibroid and night sweats.
    - Use for up to a year to see the best results for chronic issues.

Rose (Rosa ssp)

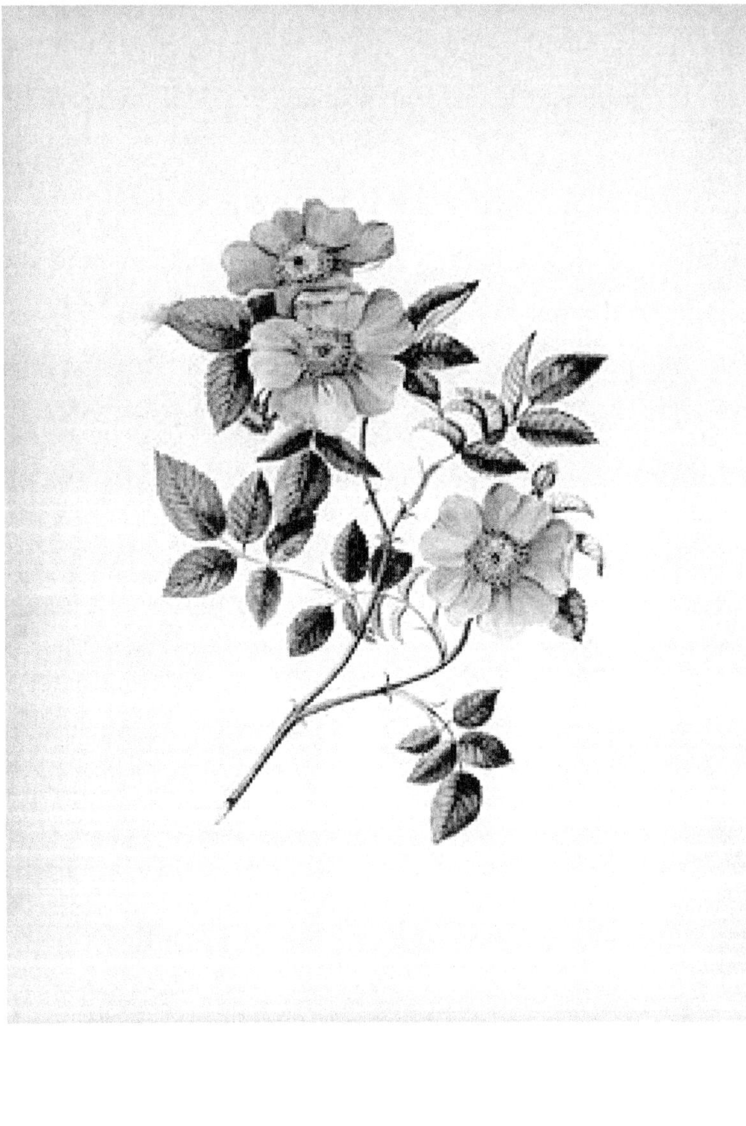

- Rose hips are often indicated for conditions where cooling, soothing, drying and/or movement are needed. In TCM rose is indicated for regulating qi, promoting circulation, and stabilizing kidneys.
- Rose is useful for high blood pressure, poor circulation, hot flashes, heart palpitations, blood tonic, pelvic congestion, scanty menses, cramps, water retention, vaginal infections, UTIs, sexual dysfunction and low libido.
- Traditionally, the Rose is known as a woman's herb. It has the ability to balance the hormones, strengthen the uterus and act as an aphrodisiac. It can be used very effectively to ease menstrual cramps internally and externally.
- Its benefits to the skin are multifaceted. It can not only balance the skin but moisturize and rejuvenate it as well. It has been used effectively in anti aging skin products for centuries.
- Containing a wide range of antioxidants, Rose petals and hips are a rich source of nutrition. Rose hips not only contain so much vitamin C that in WWII they were used as a substitute to deliver vitamin C syrup to troops in Britain, but they, along with other parts of the plant, also contain large amounts of vitamins A, B1, B2, B3, niacin, K, and E as well as polyphenols, pectin and bioflavonoids.
- Rose has the ability to open the heart and bring comfort and calming to those in need. It is incredibly uplifting and can be used to ease both depression and anxiety. It can be useful in any sort of emotional trauma, fear or stress.
- Rose is not only good for the emotional heart, but the physical heart as well. It is especially indicated in high blood pressure and/or poor circulation, and in those who experience heart palpitations and hot flashes. It also contains heart-healthy pectin.

- The petals of Rose are mucilaginous and best harvested before fully opened on a dry day.
    - Dry it for use in teas
    - Helpful for inflammation, arthritis and hemorrhoids
    - Use for depression, tension, anxiety, nervousness, anger, irritability, stress and grief

Rituals for Your Meno-Morphosis

Morning Ritual

Daily rituals are so individual that it is difficult to give examples that might resonate with every woman. However, here are a few suggestions that my clients and I have found nurturing and nourishing:

- Before rising in the morning, use a combination of energy exercises, lymphatic massage or yoga poses and stretches to wake up and energize your body and mind.
- Before getting out of bed, practice self-pleasuring with or without orgasm.
- Upon rising, light a candle to bring more intention to your morning self-care practices.
- Set your tea water to boil while you do your facial cleansing.
- When the water boils, prepare your tea to later create your Morning Energy Green Drink (pg. 176).
- Practice a few minutes of movement meditation to your favorite music, or perhaps take a short morning walk outside or visit your garden.
- Finish making your Morning Energy Green Drink and sip on it while journaling your intentions for the day.
- Blow out your candle with gratitude for the new day and the opportunities it brings.

Evening Ritual

Again, rituals are necessarily as individual as each woman and should be created to meet her unique needs. Here are a few suggestions for a soothing nighttime ritual:

- Light a candle to bring more intention to your evening self-care practices.
- Use an avocado or other replenishing facial routine.
- Perhaps luxuriate in a warm mineral salt bath and diffuse sedative essential oils or bath herbs to help you relax.
- Listen to calming music as a relaxing background to your ritual.
- Spend a few minutes in meditation with a tarot or oracle card, crystal or special relaxing herbal blend
- During menopause, creative juices can flow vividly. Keep a journal nearby during your ritual (and next to your bed if you awaken during the night) to get your inspirations out and on paper. This has the advantage of relaxing and calming the mind.
- Blow out your candle with gratitude for the day and the rest, rejuvenation and healing that the night will bring.

Full Moon Ritual

Gather your supplies:

- Altar with sacred objects you resonate with (crystals, herbs, candles), ideally outside
- Tarot or oracle card deck
- Journal, paper and pencil
- Fire pit or fire safe bowl and lighter
- Herb bundle or incense to burn
- Music or instrument such as drum or flute

Set aside some time on the evening of the full moon to be in a quiet spot where you can be undisturbed and ideally where you can see the full moon.

Prepare your space with your sacred items and light your candles if using them.

Light your incense or herb bundle and purify the space. You may want to acknowledge and honor the four directions at this time and ask that all negative energy be released and your space be protected.

Create a meditative mindset – I like to practice deep breathing and use a singing bowl. You may want to play music, drums, and so on.

Full moons are the time of releasing what no longer serves …

Draw a card from your deck with the intention of receiving guidance around what needs to be released.

Using your journal or paper, spend a few moments journaling what drops in for you.

Set your intentions for what you feel ready to release by writing them down.

When you are ready, read each intention out loud and burn the paper it is written on and watch your intention be delivered out into the universe as the smoke spirals into the sky.

To close your ritual, you may like to speak the words, "So be it!" or "It is done!" (Some say to repeat this three times) and blow out your candle.

You may wish to remain in your space and journal any inspiration that comes up after your ritual.

New Moon Ritual

Gather your supplies:

- Altar with sacred objects you resonate with (crystals, herbs, candles) ideally outside
- Tarot or oracle card deck
- Journal, paper and pencil
- Fire pit or fire safe bowl and lighter
- Herb bundle or incense to burn
- Music or instrument such as drum or flute

Set aside some time on the evening of the new moon to be in a quiet spot where you can be undisturbed.

Prepare your space with your sacred items and light your candles if using them.

Light your incense or herb bundle and purify the space. You may want to acknowledge and honor the four directions at this time and ask that all negative energy be released and your space be protected.

Create a meditative mindset – I like to practice deep breathing and use a singing bowl. You may want to play music, drums, and so on.

New moons are the time for setting new intentions and new

beginnings …

Draw a card from your deck with the intention of receiving guidance around what to focus on to bring your new intention into being.

Using your journal or paper, spend a few moments journaling what drops in for you.

Set your intentions for what you feel ready to birth into the world by writing them down.

When you are ready, read each intention out loud and burn the paper it is written on and watch your intention be delivered out into the universe as the smoke spirals into the sky.

To close your ritual, you may like to speak the words, "So be it!" or "It is done!" (Some say to repeat this three times) and blow out your candle.

You may wish to remain in your space and journal any inspiration that comes up after your ritual.

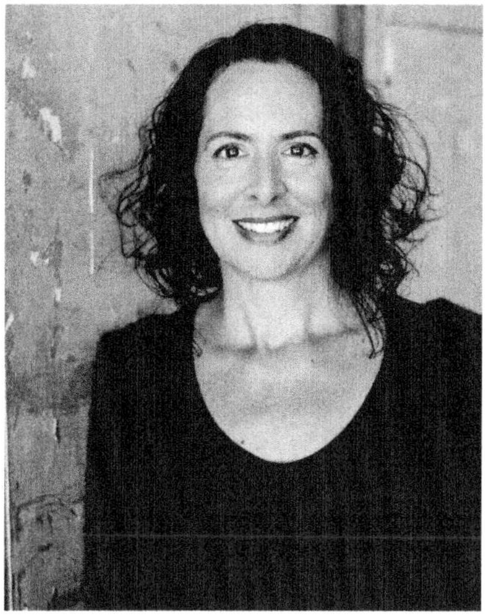

About Vanessa

As a Traditional Naturopath, Vanessa Nixon is passionate about helping women thrive during the spiritual initiation of their menopausal journey. She is adept at attunement to natural health, invigorating dance and therapeutic movement, and teaching women to see their innate natural beauty.

After reimagining her life at age 50, Vanessa discovered a profound and deeply intuitive process that helped her to embrace her fabulous inner wise woman fearlessly. She now shares these powerful and ancient initiations with women in the US and beyond who want to reclaim vibrant good health in their own sacred mid-life transit.

Vanessa Nixon lives in the Pacific Northwest and is CEO of the natural cosmetics company, Natural Look Mineral Make-Up. When she is not practicing in the realm of natural health and organic beauty, she is a professional Belly Dance instructor.

Professional credentials:

Doctorate in Traditional Naturopathy

Master's in Herbal Medicine

Certificate in Aromatherapy

Certificate in Homeopathy

Certificate in Iridology

Certificate in Nutrition

Certificate in Reflexology

Professional Middle Eastern Dance Performer and Instructor

Founder and CEO of Natural Look Mineral Makeup

Vanessa's online resources:

- Websites – https://www.herbsofgracehealingarts.com/ https://www.herbsofgrace.com/
- FB Group – You Can Feel Marvelous in Midlife, Naturally! https://www.facebook.com/groups/797232817813731
- FB Page – https://www.facebook.com/HerbsofGraceHealingArts

- Insta – https://www.instagram.com/herbsofgrace/
- LinkedIn – https://www.linkedin.com/in/vanessa-nixon/
- Twitter – https://twitter.com/HerbsofGrace

Vanessa's Program links:

- https://www.herbsofgracehealingarts.com/vibrant-mid-life-immersion
- https://www.herbsofgracehealingarts.com/bellydancing-thru-life-membership
- https://vanessa-nixon.xperiencify.io/

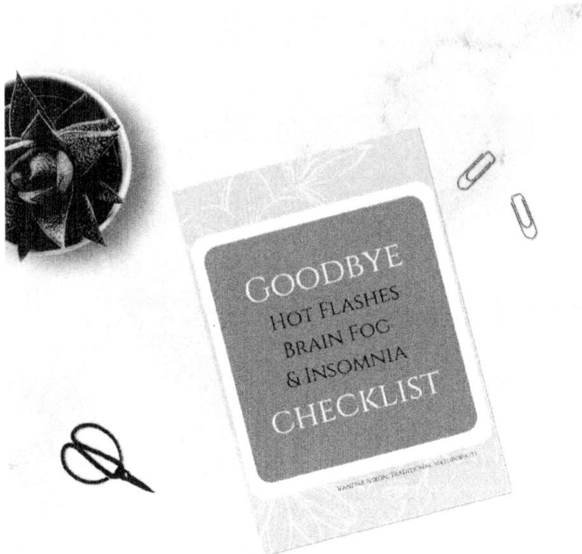

Your Free Gift

"Goodbye Hot Flashes, Brain Fog & Insomnia Checklist" is a FREE resource I've created for women navigating midlife. Reduce your menopause symptoms naturally as you step into the most powerful chapter of your life.

Go here https://www.herbsofgracehealingarts.com/free-checklist to grab this handy and useful tool

Empower your midlife journey today!